Working Memory in the Primary

This highly practical resource has been designed to support working memory and curriculum success in the Key Stage 1 and Key Stage 2 classroom. Working memory is crucial for success in maths, reading, reading comprehension and problem solving, yet children with poor working memory often struggle to meet the demands of everyday classroom activities.

Filled with activities and support for Key Stage 1 and Key Stage 2 Maths and English, this book offers ideas for the practising teacher on how to make the classroom a place to reinforce memory skills, and to ensure that those with working memory difficulties are included and supported.

Key features include:

- Information on recognising working memory difficulties
- Practical and specific strategies to support learners in the classroom
- Graduated activities for Maths and English learners based on the national curriculum

The importance of working memory on curriculum success is becoming increasingly evident, with growing emphasis on testing and an ever more demanding curriculum. With photocopiable and downloadable resources, this is an essential book for teachers, teaching assistants and other education staff looking to support working memory with children.

Catherine Routley has worked for over 25 years in the field of special needs, supporting individual children and developing training courses for learning support assistants and teachers.

WORKING MEMORY IN THE PRIMARY CLASSROOM

Practical and Inclusive Strategies for Curriculum Success in Maths and English

CATHERINE ROUTLEY

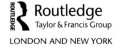

Routledge
Taylor & Francis Group

LONDON AND NEW YORK

First published 2021
by Routledge
2 Park Square, Milton Park, Abingdon, Oxon OX14 4RN

and by Routledge
52 Vanderbilt Avenue, New York, NY 10017

Routledge is an imprint of the Taylor & Francis Group, an informa business

British Library Cataloguing-in-Publication Data
A catalogue record for this book is available from the British Library

Library of Congress Cataloging-in-Publication Data
Names: Routley, Catherine, author.
Title: Working memory in the primary classroom : practical and inclusive strategies for curriculum success / Catherine Routley.
Description: Abingdon, Oxon ; New York, NY : Routledge, 2021.
Identifiers: LCCN 2020029591 (print) | LCCN 2020029592 (ebook) | ISBN 9780367567125 (hardback) | ISBN 9780367416980 (paperback) | ISBN 9780367814342 (ebook)
Subjects: LCSH: Learning disabled children—Education (Primary) | Short-term memory. | Education, Primary—Curricula.
Classification: LCC LC4704.73 .R68 2021 (print) | LCC LC4704.73 (ebook) | DDC 371.9/0472—dc23
LC record available at https://lccn.loc.gov/2020029591
LC ebook record available at https://lccn.loc.gov/2020029592

ISBN: 978-0-367-56712-5 (hbk)
ISBN: 978-0-367-41698-0 (pbk)
ISBN: 978-0-367-81434-2 (ebk)

Typeset in Univers LT Std
by KnowledgeWorks Global Ltd.

Visit the companion website: www.routledge.com/cw/speechmark

Contents

CONTENTS

Introduction

Some notes on the curriculum and working memory

There is an increasing body of evidence, which suggests that working memory is linked to effective learning, a view emphasised by many researchers in this field, in particular Gathercole et al 2004, 2008.

Evidence of working memory problems has been found in individuals with reading and maths difficulties, language impairments, hearing impairment and Attention Deficit/Hyperactivity Disorder (ADHD).

Those of us at the 'coal face' of education hold the view that the national curriculum is being implemented at a fast rate and places considerable demands on all children. Children with poor working memory often struggle to meet the heavy demands of everyday classroom activities because they are unable to hold sufficient information in their minds to allow task completion. They are also asked to hold information whilst engaged in other activities, causing memory overload, which has a negative impact on the pupils' working memory function. Coupled with the amount of information needing to be retained, the environment of the classroom offers distractions, both visual and oral, which again have an adverse effect on working memory.

There is a body of evidence which suggests poor working memory is occurring in all pupils, not necessarily those with Special Educational Needs and Disability (SEND). There are reports linking dependence on technology (smart phones) by primary age children as having a detrimental impact on their working memory – Why try to work things out when it's done for you so quickly by your phone/computer?

Although we look to working memory as being crucial to Maths and English success, there are other roles it plays in learning: making connections between temporary storage and manipulation of the information necessary for such complex cognitive tasks as language, comprehension, learning and reasoning.

Working memory is a skill which is essential for accessing the curriculum efficiently and at the same time it is one which is deteriorating. Various reasons have been suggested for this decline: predominantly the increased use of technology which now begins from a very young age. Amongst the crowded curriculum is there a space for sessions on working memory – exercises to improve this much needed skill? Possibly not but it cannot be denied.

This book is not one which is totally comprehensive of the content of the National Curriculum, but it is one which offers strategies as to the majority of the basic learning required.

General classroom strategies to help pupils with working memory difficulty

Individual memory aids:

Number line 0 – 100

Keywords and facts relating to the current topic, i.e. properties of shape, positional language

Examples of sentence starters

Mnemonics for remembering information, i.e. position of planets in relation to the earth

> My very eager mother just served us nachos

> (Mercury, Venus, Earth, Mars, Jupiter, Saturn, Uranus, Neptune)

Mind map focusing on the main idea of the story

Examples and definitions of adverbs/vocabulary to be used during the lesson

Maths vocabulary and formula for, i.e. area, perimeter

CPS reminder (capital letters, punctuation and sentences)

As we all learn differently, not all memory aids will be suitable for all children. Children need to be shown a range of strategies before they can evaluate which works best for them. They also need to develop skills in devising their own memory aids so they can start using them independently and it becomes part of their learning process.

Teaching strategies

Important points to remember:

- Always put memory aids on children's table where they are working – they will rarely look around the room for information

- Provide visuals – make print from handouts in a larger font always, incorporate visuals
- Do not put too much information on a handout – it's preferable to give additional sheets rather than overload one page
- Always relate new information to that already learned
- Reinforce previously learned facts
- Present new information in the middle of the lesson
- Use visuals to learn new vocabulary, i.e. Uneasy (worried, anxious) Roger the rabbit feels uneasy when Sammy the snake squeezes
- Provide concrete aids such as unfix cubes to remind pupil there are three parts to the instruction

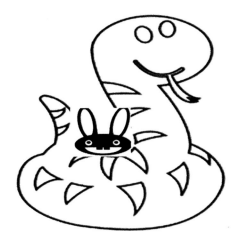

- Remember to reduce memory overload, avoid giving lengthy instructions and unfamiliar content Provide a distraction-free environment as much as possible – always close the door, use 'traffic lights' to reduce classroom noise
- Encourage the children to develop their own strategies
- Provide extra time for processing of language
- Provide information in chunks
- Provide opportunities to repeat the instructions/tasks
- Encourage checking work for: *CPS*
- *Capital letters*: (Have I made sure all proper nouns, beginning of sentences start with a capital letters?)
- *Punctuation*: (Have I put the right punctuation at the end of each sentence? Such as ? ! . " " : ; ,)
- *Sentences*: (Have I used proper sentences, can my handwriting be easily read, if necessary, have I asked for help?)

How to spot a pupil with working memory problems

Does he/she:

- Have a short attention span?

- Lose their place in complicated tasks and/or when counting?

- Appear to not be paying attention or easily distracted?

- Fail to complete assignments?

- Forget how to complete an activity that has been started, even when it has been clearly explained?

- Put hand up to answer questions but can't remember what they were going to say?

- Fail to complete common classroom activities that require large amounts of information to be held in memory?

- Display incomplete recall of information or events?

- Benefit from continued teacher support during lengthy activities?

- Need a neighbour to remind them of the task in hand?

- Find group activities difficult, rarely participates?

- Sequence oral information incorrectly?

- Demonstrate poor academic progress, particularly in reading and maths?

- Find copying from the board difficult?

- Have difficulty following multi-step directions. Forget part(s) and tend to remember last instruction only?

Key Stage 1 - Maths

Early numbers

Numbers 1 to 5

Remember 0 means nothing

1   One howling wolf $1 + 0 = 1$ $0 + 1 = 1$

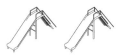

2   Two slippery slides $2 + 0 = 2$ $1 + 1 = 2$

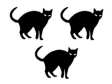

3   Three curious cats $3 + 0 = 3$ $2 + 1 = 3$

$0 + 3 = 3$ $1 + 2 = 3$

4   Four friendly mice $4 + 0 = 4$ $3 + 1 = 4$

$2 + 2 = 4$ $0 + 4 = 4$ $1 + 3 = 4$

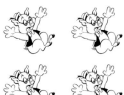

5   Five flying pigs $5 + 0 = 5$ $4 + 1 = 5$ $3 + 2 = 5$

$0 + 5 = 5$ $1 + 4 = 5$ $2 + 3 = 5$

Can you tell me what 1 + 1 make?   Can you tell me what 2 + 1 make?

Can you tell me what 4 + 1 make?   Can you tell me 2 ways of making 5?

Can you tell me 3 ways of making 3?

2 numbers that make 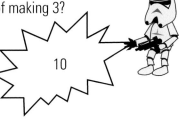 10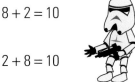

10 + 0 = 10   9 + 1 = 10   8 + 2 = 10

0 + 10 = 10   1 + 9 = 10   2 + 8 = 10

7 + 3 = 10   6 + 4 = 10   5 + 5 = 10

3 + 7 = 10   4 + 6 = 10

Match up the numbers to make 5

2   1

5   3

3   2

4   0

0   5

What do you need to make 10? Work out the missing numbers

$7 + ? = 10$ $8 + ? = 10$ $6 + ? = 10$ $5 + ? = 10$ $10 + ? = 10$

$5 + 4 + ? = 10$ $2 + 1 + ? = 10$ $6 + 2 + ? = 10$ $8 + 1 + ? = 10$

$2 + ? + 5$ $4 + ? = 5$

Counting in 2s to 10

Benny Bean loves taking giant steps. He wants to step over the rocks so he can count in 2s to 10. Can you count in 2s?

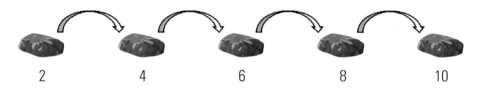

2   4   6   8   10

Draw more birds in the box to make 5

Draw more smiley faces in the box to make 7

☺ ☺ ☺

Draw more lollipops in the box to make 9

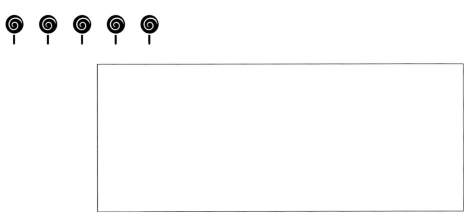

Draw more stars in the box to make 10

★ ★ ★ ★ ★ ★
★ ★

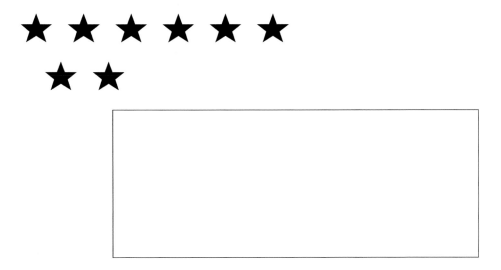

Using a number line

Harry Hare is out hunting for dinosaurs. But he is not that good at numbers, so he needs a number line and your help.

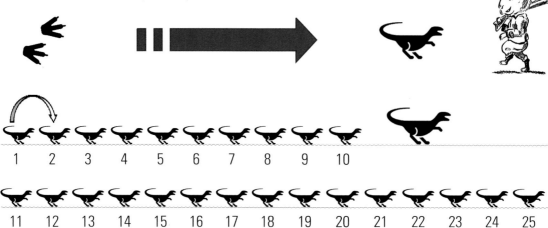

| 1 | 2 | 3 | 4 | 5 | 6 | 7 | 8 | 9 | 10 |

| 11 | 12 | 13 | 14 | 15 | 16 | 17 | 18 | 19 | 20 | 21 | 22 | 23 | 24 | 25 |

What number is 1 more than 14?

What number is 2 more than 15?

What number is 4 more than 16?

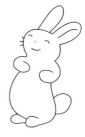

What number is 3 more than 18?

What number is 2 more than 12?

Now, eyes shut like Rod the rabbit, no looking at the number line

Can you tell me the number which is 2 more than 12?

What number is 2 more than 17?

What is the number 2 more than 16?

What is the number 1 more than 18?

What is the number 2 more than 17?

Can you count in 2s to 10 putting the numbers on the box numbers on the boxes?

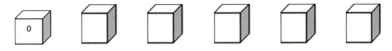

Counting in 2s and 5s

Counting in 2s to 20

Froggy has hopped over the numbers so he can count in 2s. *Using Froggy can you count in 2s to 20?*

1	2	3	4	5	6	7	8	9	10
11	12	13	14	15	16	17	18	19	20

Can you put in the missing numbers in Froggy's number line?

2 ＿＿ 6 ＿＿ 10 ＿＿ 14 ＿＿ ＿＿ 20

Can you count in 2s from 2 to 10 with your eyes shut? Now can you count from 10 to 20?

Counting in 5s

1	2	3	4	5	6	7	8	9	10
11	12	13	14	15	16	17	18	19	20
21	22	23	24	25	26	27	28	29	30
31	32	33	34	35	36	37	38	39	40
41	42	43	44	45	46	47	48	49	50

Practise counting in 5s

Now I will say 5 and you say _____ I will say 15 and you say _____ I will say 25, your turn _____
My turn 35, your turn _____ My turn 45, your turn _____ .

Now backwards, I will say 50, your turn _____ I say 40, your turn _____ I say 30, your turn _____
I say 20, your turn _____ I say 10, your turn _____

Can you fill in the missing numbers?

5, ___ 15, ___ , ___ , 30, ___ 40, ___ , 50   0, ___ , ___ , ___ , 20   10, 15, 20, ___ , ___ ,

___ , ___ , ___ , 50 ,   20, ___ , ___ , ___ 40   15, ___ , ___ , ___ , ___ , 40, ___ , 50

Counting on: making the number bigger. To the right, numbers get bigger. More than = bigger

⟹

1 2 3 4 5 6 7 8 9 10 11 12 13 14 15 16 17 18 19 20 21 22 23 24 25 30 30 35 40 45 50

Using your pointing finger:

Can you count on 3 from 9? The answer is . . . .

Can you count 5 on from 12?   The answer is . . . .

Can you count on 5 from 45?   It's . . . .

I counted 4 on from 17 and it's . . . .

I think counting 6 on from 11 is 18. Am I right?

Counting 3 on from 27 is . . . .

I counted on 6 from 17 and I think it's 24. Am I right?

Making 20 baby dinosaurs, Dino will be your guide showing you some ways to make 20

$9 + 11 = 20$ $20 + 0 = 20$ $7 + 13 = 20$ $10 + 10 = 20$

$5 + 15 = 20$ $18 + 2 = 20$ $4 + 16 = 20$

Here are some more sums which add up to 20

Do these sums add up to 20?

$6 + 14 = 20$ $12 + 8 = 20$ $16 + 4 = 20$ $20 + 4 = ?$ $17 + 7 = ?$ $18 + 6 = ?$

Work out the missing numbers:

$2 + ? = 20$ $20 + ? = 20$ $3 + ? = 20$ $? + 19 = 20$

Now ... counting in 10s

It's so easy, it's like the numbers 1 to 10 with a zero stuck on the end

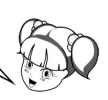

| 0 | 10 | 20 | 30 | 40 | 50 | 60 | 70 | 80 | 90 | 100 |

Jason the crafty cat wants the birds to help him counting in 10x

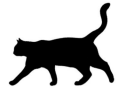

Can you fill in the missing 10s?

0 _____, 20, _____, 40, _____, 60, _____, 80, _____, 100

0, 5, _____, 15, _____, _____, 30, _____, _____, 45, _____, 55, _____, 65, _____, 75

More missing numbers

0, 2, 4, _____, _____, _____, _____, _____.

68, 70, _____, _____, _____, _____, 80, _____.

18, _____, _____, _____, _____, 28, _____, _____.

24, _____, _____, _____, _____, 34, 36, _____.

15 _____, 25 _____, _____, _____, 45, _____, 55.

20, _____, _____, 50, _____, 70, _____, 90, _____.

Counting in 10s using cubes

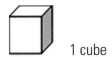 1 cube

10 cubes altogether make 1 ten

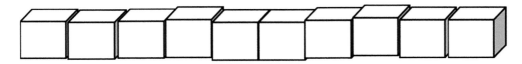

Each line has 10 blocks   What numbers are these?

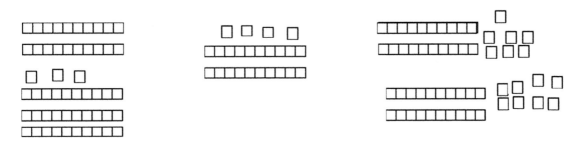

Draw this number block using the right number of tens and ones for   27   43   38   45   50   15   37

Writing numbers

0 zero	5 five
1 one	6 six
2 two	7 seven
3 three	8 eight
4 four	9 nine

The numbers above have only one number and are called single digits. Two-digit numbers start from ten:

10 ten

11 eleven

12 twelve

These are two-digit numbers, they all have 1 digit in the tens column and 1 digit in the ones column.

The Teens

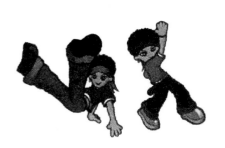

13 thirteen   16 sixteen

14 fourteen   17 seventeen

15 fifteen   18 eighteen

19 nineteen

Different numbers of tens have different words

Twenty 20   Fifty 50   Eighty 80

Thirty 30   Sixty 60   Ninety 90

Forty 40   Seventy 70

Can you write these numbers in words?

16   0   5   16   18   2   3   13

To write the numbers after 19, you write the tens bit first then the ones

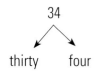

34

thirty   four

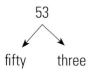

53

fifty   three

Can you write these numbers in words?

44   52   35   23   61   22   34

Putting numbers in order

Put these in order from smallest number to the biggest

6   5   7   2   0   10   20

That's easy
I think....

Look at these double-digit numbers

57   84   32   71

How do you put them in order from smallest to biggest?

Look at the numbers, the tens first, which is the smallest?

You have   5   8   3   7   putting them in order smallest to biggest:

3   5   7   8

Now look at the numbers next to them, the ones   7   4   3   1

The answer is   32   57   71   84

Look at the numbers, the tens first, which tens is the smallest and goes first? You know 8 is the biggest so it goes last and there are two numbers in between.

Look at these numbers

43   22   53   47   24

If the numbers have the same tens but different ones, then you put the smallest ones first.

There are two numbers with 2 tens: 22 and 24

Which has the smallest number of ones? So, 22 goes first

	T	O
	2	2
	2	4

There are two numbers both with 4 lots of tens, which one is the smallest?

Now look at the ones It's 42, so it goes before 47

22 24 42 47 53

Can you put these numbers in sequence (the right order) from smallest to biggest?

5   20   7   8   15   2   0   34   25   10   8   19   9

55   42   40   27   34   30   67   33   16   24   61   30

Can you write these words as numbers?

Thirteen   Twenty   Sixteen   Ten   Zero   Twelve   Thirty   Forty-Five   Fifty

Ordinal numbers

Don't worry it's just another word for first, 1st, second, 2nd, third 3rd, fourth, 4th, ...

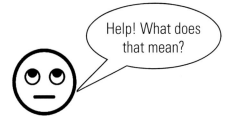

  Sam won the race. He came first, 1st

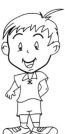

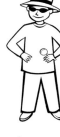

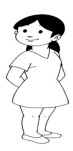

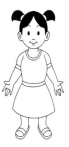

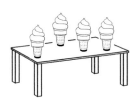

4th Fourth   3rd Third   2nd Second   1st First

The children are queuing for ice cream at the school fair. Karen is first in the queue, Sita second, Karl is third and Mikal is fourth. There is no one after Mikal, so he is **last** in the queue.

*Put a line under the car which is **last** in the line at the traffic lights.*

*Put a line under the car which is **second** at the traffic lights.*

Four hungry dogs, underline (a) the third one to get his food, (b) the fourth and (c) the first.

Adding

John has 3 sweets

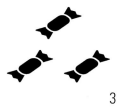

3

Peter has 4 sweets

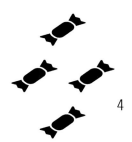

4

Altogether they have 7 sweets

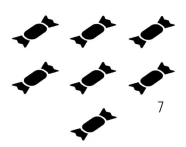

7

Jane has 5 teddies

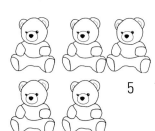

5

Kate has 3 teddies

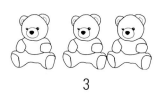

3

Altogether they have 8 teddies

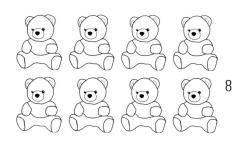

8

Here are 6 toy robots

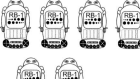

6

Here are 4 more

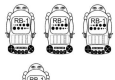

4

How many altogether?

Some more adding

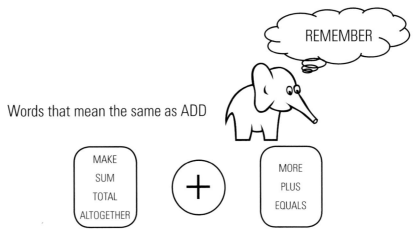

Words that mean the same as ADD

MAKE
SUM
TOTAL
ALTOGETHER

$+$

MORE
PLUS
EQUALS

Adding together. *Try these sums.*

$4 + 5 =$	$5 + 5 =$	$5 + 7 =$	$10 + 9 =$
$9 + 8 =$	$15 + 5 =$	$6 + 11 =$	$13 + 0 =$
$14 + 3 =$	$11 + 5 =$	$20 + 11 =$	$30 + 5 =$

Can you work out the answers?

Two and two makes …   Four plus six …   Five more than ten …   Five and five equals …

The total of two and six …   Eight and two …   The sum of seven and five …   Seven and five total …

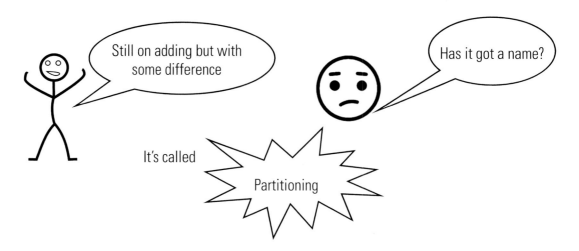

It's called

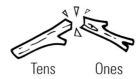

Partitioning means splitting or breaking the numbers into tens and ones before adding them together.

Tens   Ones

Partition (split) the numbers into tens and ones

12 means 1 ten and 2 ones

24 means there are 2 tens and 4 ones

48 means there are 4 tens and 8 ones

Here's an example

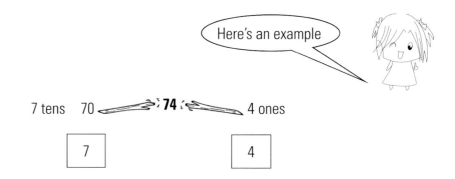

7 tens   70 → **74** ← 4 ones

| 7 | | 4 |

Can you use partitioning to break up these numbers?   37   49   78   97

Adding problems: Underline the important words to do the sum

Peter has 4 sweets and Katie has 5. How many do they have altogether?

Jacob ran 6 miles on Friday and 7 miles on Saturday. What is the total of miles he ran?

Jennifer ate 3 pieces of toast on Monday and on Tuesday. How many did she eat altogether?

Steph ate 3 ice creams on Saturday, 2 on Sunday and 1 on Monday. What is the sum of the ice creams Steph ate?

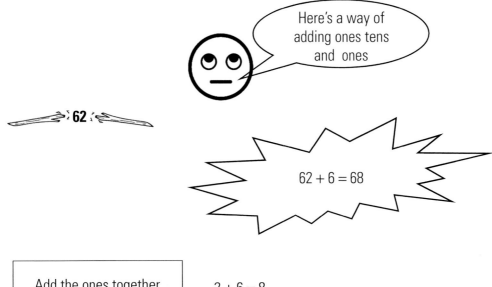

$62 + 6$ | Add the ones together | $2 + 6 = 8$

Add the tens $= 1 + 6 = 7$

Add the ones $0 + 6 = 6$ Answer 76

$16 + 60$ $16 = 1$ ten $+ 6$ ones

$60 = 6$ tens and 0 one

Add the tens together

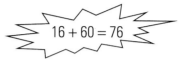

$16 + 60 = 76$

Use partitioning to add both numbers   T   O

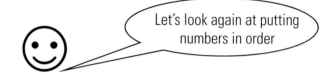

$54 = 50 + 4$ $25 = 20 + 5$

$54 = 50 + 4$

$25 = 20 + 5$

$79 = 70 + 9$

Use partitioning to add these numbers: $53 + 72$ $37 + 12$ $33 + 42$ $63 + 43$

☺ Let's look again at putting numbers in order

How do we put   78   27   34   75   in order starting with the smallest?

27 has the smallest amount of tens (2) so it goes **first**, 34 has the next smallest number of tens (3)

27   34

We now have two numbers 78 and 75 with the same number in the tens, so what do we do?

We look at the next number, the ones number which is the smallest it's ... 75, so we have 78 left. So 75 is smaller than 78.

Look at these numbers. Can you put the *smallest* first?

40   32   33   67   69   49   18   39   63   66

Can you put the *biggest* number first?

37   88   54   2   60   34   89   33   5   12   67   80   44   42   3

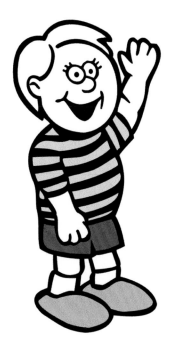

Something New
SUBTRACTION

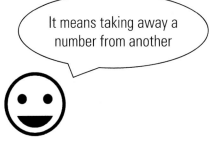

It means taking away a number from another

There are 4 cakes

Jacki takes 1 of them

There are 3 cakes left

4 − 1 = 3 The sign for subtraction (take away) is —

Oh dear! Our dinosaur has become very fierce. It's running away time!

Using your <u>number line</u> to subtract, remember the numbers get smaller

0 1 2 3 4 5 6 7 8 9 10 11 12 13 14 15 16 17 18 19 20 21 22 23 24 25

Use your number line to work out: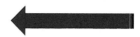

What is 10 take away 2   5 take away 3   7 take away 4

Use the number line to find the answers: $10 - 6 =$ $15 - 3 =$ $21 - 5 =$ $22 - 4 =$

Words that mean the same as subtraction $(-)$

Take away

Remainder

What is the difference?

Fewer

Minus

Decrease

Less

Left

What is the difference?

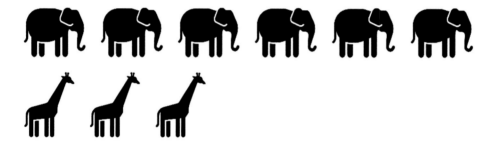

6 elephants

3 giraffes

Using subtraction to find the difference between the number of elephants and the number of giraffes. Patrik has finished these sums, now it's your turn to have a go.

Subtraction sums

$13 - 10 = 3$ $10 - 3 = 7$ $18 - 4 = 14$ $16 - 8 = 8$ $9 - 5 = 4$

$10 - 4 =$ $18 - 6 =$ $22 - 5 =$ $25 - 8 =$ $19 - 9 =$ $23 - 7 =$

What is the answer?

15 less 10   8 less 2   7 minus 3   8 minus 3

The difference between 15 and 8

Decrease 19 by 9 what is left?

I take 11 from 15 what is left?

Problems using subtraction: Remember to underline the words you need to find the answers

Mark was given 5 bars of chocolate, but he ate 3, how many has he got left?

Salim had 5 fish fingers, but he only ate 2, how many fish fingers were left?

Jane was given 10 presents for her birthday, but she gave 2 to her friend, how many fewer presents has she got now?

Delia bought 7 packs of stickers and gave 2 to Maddy, how many are left for her?

There were 10 footballs in the sports cupboard, 7 were lent to class, how many remain in the cupboard?

Grouping

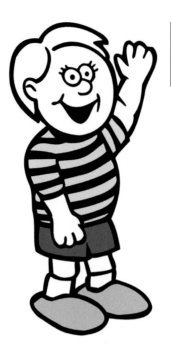

Something new
GROUPING

How many spaceship models does Peter Have? He has 3 groups of 2 models OR 3 groups of 3.

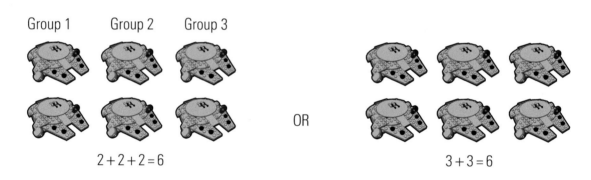

Group 1   Group 2   Group 3

$2 + 2 + 2 = 6$ OR $3 + 3 = 6$

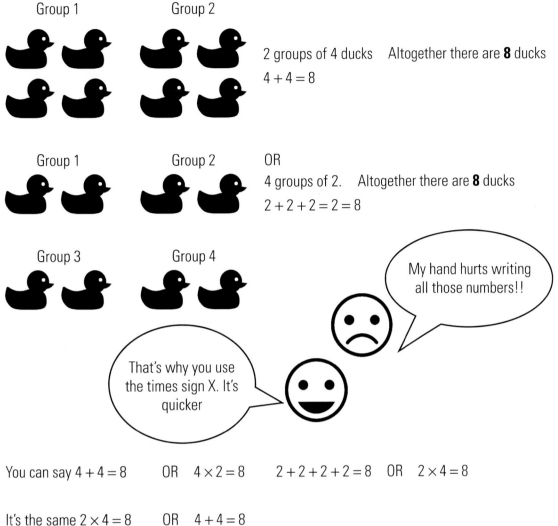

Group 1   Group 2

2 groups of 4 ducks   Altogether there are **8** ducks

$4 + 4 = 8$

Group 1   Group 2   OR

4 groups of 2.   Altogether there are **8** ducks

$2 + 2 + 2 = 2 = 8$

Group 3   Group 4

My hand hurts writing all those numbers!!

That's why you use the times sign X. It's quicker

You can say $4 + 4 = 8$ OR $4 \times 2 = 8$ $2 + 2 + 2 + 2 = 8$ OR $2 \times 4 = 8$

It's the same $2 \times 4 = 8$ OR $4 + 4 = 8$

Use **multiplication to** find the total number of doughnuts

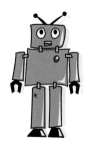

Another world for grouping is

MULTIPLICATION

Altogether there are 10 doughnuts in these groups of 5 $5 \times 2 = 10$

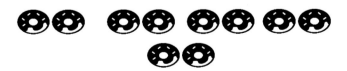

Can you group them in a different way and get the same answer?

Can you show 2 ways of grouping the ice lollies to get the same answer?

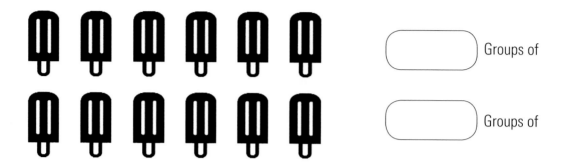

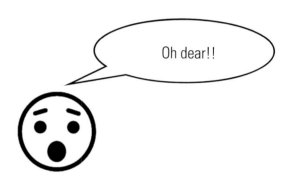

Groups of

Groups of

Times tables have to be learned!

Oh dear!!

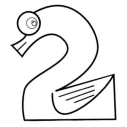

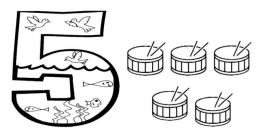

2 × 1 ⇨ 2

2 × 2 ⇨ 4

2 × 3 ⇨ 6

2 × 4 ⇨ 8

2 × 5 ⇨ 10

2 × 6 ⇨ 12

2 × 7 ⇨ 14

2 × 8 ⇨ 16

2 × 9 ⇨ 18

2 × 10 ⇨ 20

2 × 11 ⇨ 22

2 × 12 ⇨ 24

5 × 1 ⇨ 5

5 × 2 ⇨ 10

5 × 3 ⇨ 15

5 × 4 ⇨ 20

5 × 5 ⇨ 25

5 × 6 ⇨ 30

5 × 7 ⇨ 35

5 × 8 ⇨ 40

5 × 9 ⇨ 45

5 × 10 ⇨ 50

5 × 11 ⇨ 55

5 × 12 ⇨ 60

Why is the 10 (ten) times table the easiest to remember?

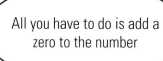

All you have to do is add a zero to the number

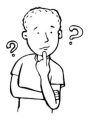

$10 \times 6 = 60$ $10 \times 5 = 50$ $10 \times 10 = 100$ $10 \times 2 = 20$ $10 \times 4 = 40$ $10 \times 7 = 70$

$10 \times 8 = 80$ $10 \times 9 = 90$ $10 \times 11 = 110$ $10 \times 4 = 40$ $10 \times 3 = 30$ $10 \times 12 = 120$

Can you work out these sums?

$10 \times 2 =$ $10 \times 3 =$ $10 \times 8 =$ $10 \times 9 =$

$10 \times 12 =$ $10 \times 0 =$ $5 \times 5 =$ $2 \times 8 =$

$10 \times 5 =$ $5 \times 4 =$ $2 \times 7 =$ $10 \times 10 =$

$5 \times 9 =$ $2 \times 3 =$ $2 \times 9 =$ $10 \times 8 =$

Some problems with multiplication:

Jane has 5 pencil pots, each one has 4 pencils.
How many pencils altogether?

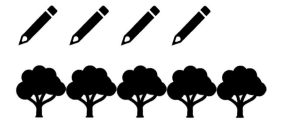

There are 5 trees and each one has 7 apples on it.
How many apples altogether?

Can you underline the multiplications in the circles which both equal 10?

1×10
2×6

1×5
10×2

0×10
5×5

2×6
2×9

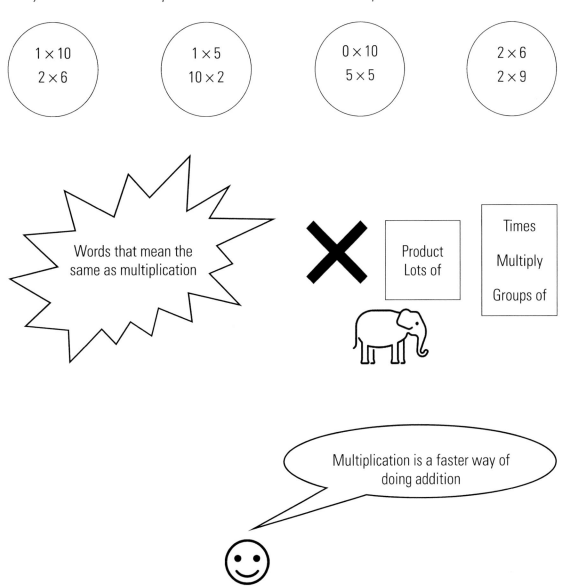

Words that mean the same as multiplication

Product
Lots of

Times

Multiply

Groups of

Multiplication is a faster way of doing addition

Shapes

We see them all around.

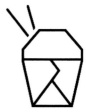
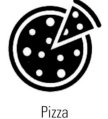

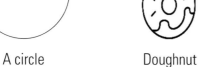
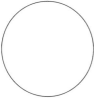

A circle	Doughnut	Clock	Pizza

A circle is a **curved** shape, it has no **edges**.

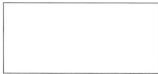

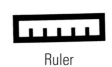

A rectangle	Television	Suitcase	Ruler

A rectangle has **four** straight sides, the **two** faces are the same length.

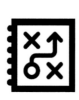
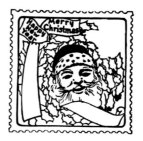
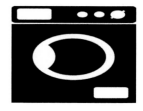

A square	Book	Stamp	Washing machine

A square has four straight sides, **all** are of the same length.

Fractions (a part of something)

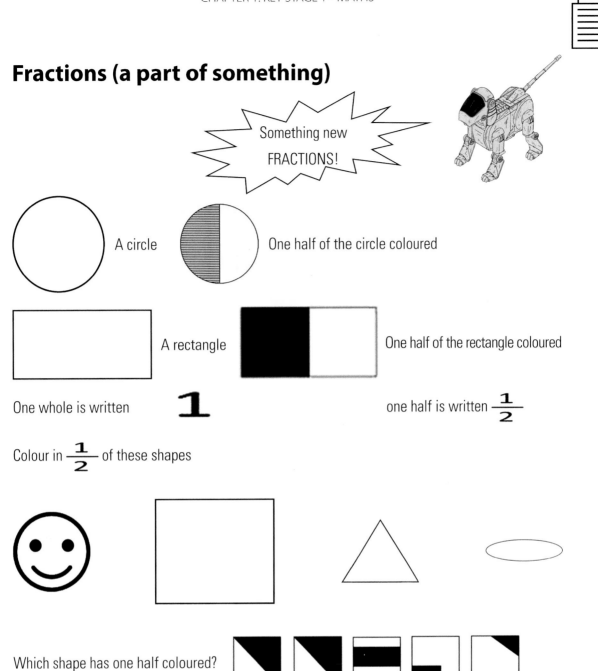

Something new
FRACTIONS!

A circle

One half of the circle coloured

A rectangle

One half of the rectangle coloured

One whole is written **1**

one half is written $\frac{1}{2}$

Colour in $\frac{1}{2}$ of these shapes

Which shape has one half coloured?

Long and short

The snake is long

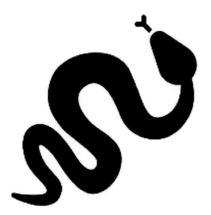

The fence is long

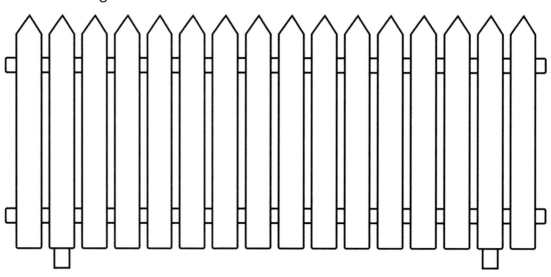

The opposite of long is short

The caterpillar is short

The pencil is short

You can match up sizes and find out which is the longer or shorter by **comparing one against the other**.

Pete's boat is **shorter** than Bill's

Pete's boat

Bill's boat

Mrs. Green's fence

Mrs. White's fence

Mrs. White's fence is **shorter** than Mrs. Green's

Who has the **longer** ruler?

Patrik's ruler

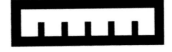

Jason' s ruler

Who has the **shorter** pencil?

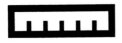

Jacob

Matthew

Heights

When you're talking about heights, they can be **tall** or **short**.

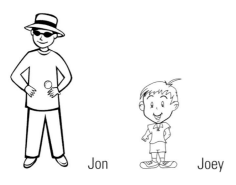

Jon   Joey

You can compare heights the same way as you can compare long and short.

Jon is **taller** than Joey.

Which one is shorter? The rabbit or the giraffe?

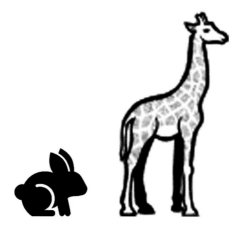

Can you draw two houses and make one taller?

Draw two flowers and make one shorter.

Something new

MEASURING ….

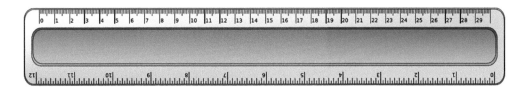

We measure in **centimetres** you can see on this ruler. It is important to measure accurately (that means properly).

Use your ruler to measure the tree and the door.

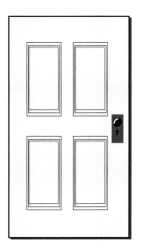

The tree measures ……cms (that's how to write centimetres easily)   The door measures ……cms

Money

Coins we use

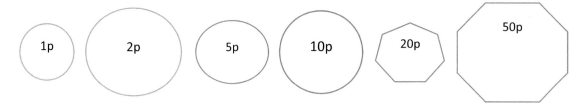

This apple costs 50p   Draw the coin I need

This lolly cost 20p   Draw the coin I need

1 ice cream costs 5p   I want to buy 2. Draw the coin or coins I need

How much does 1 slice of cake cost?   10p   5p

How much do these bananas cost?

20p   2p

Don't forget you are adding money
Remember the pence sign (p)

Try these money adding sums

20p + 10p =   50p + 1p =   1p + 20p =   10p + 2p =

20p + 20p =   10p + 5p =   20p + 30p =

Money problems

Jez buys a drink and lollipop. How much has he spent?

  50p   20p

Chris buys a pencil for 40p, a rubber for 20p. How much has he spent?

Finn buys 2 books, 1 for 50p and 1 for 40p. How much do they cost altogether?

Philip wants to buy 1 lollipop for 15p. He has 20p, does he have enough?

Petra buys 3 slices of cake, each cost 25p. How much has she spent?

Jacob has 55p. Has he got enough to buy 2 ice creams that cost 30p each?

Mo has 50p. He has bought a drink for 20p. How much has he got left?

Theo has 60p. How much will he have left if he buys 2 books that cost 20p each?

Days of the week

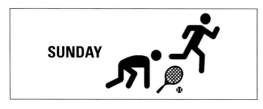

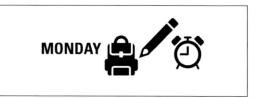

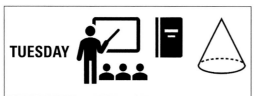

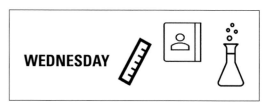

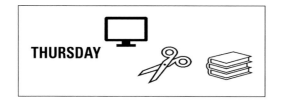

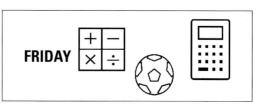

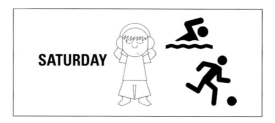

When we say TODAY it means NOW

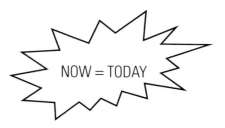

NOW = TODAY

YESTERDAY is the day **BEFORE** today.

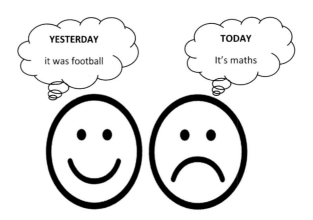

Today is **Monday** so **Sunday** is the day before, it's finished so it is going **back**

Sunday

Monday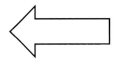

Tuesday

Wednesday   Today is Wednesday, the day before (back) is Tuesday

Thursday

Friday   Today is Friday, the day before is Thursday

Saturday   Today is Saturday, the day before is Friday

The day before Thursday is ......   The day before Saturday is ......

The day before Wednesday is ......   The day before Tuesday is ......

TOMORROW is the day **AFTER** today, you go **forwards** (it has not happened yet)

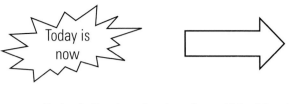

Sunday   Today is Sunday, the day after will be Monday

Monday

Tuesday

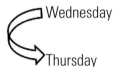Wednesday   Today is Wednesday, the day after will be Thursday

Thursday

Friday   Today is Friday, the day after will be Saturday

Saturday

The day after Tuesday will be ......

The day after Thursday will be ......

The day after Saturday will be ......

The day after Monday will be ......

The day after Sunday will be ......

The day after Friday will be ......

The day after Wednesday will be ......

Months of the year

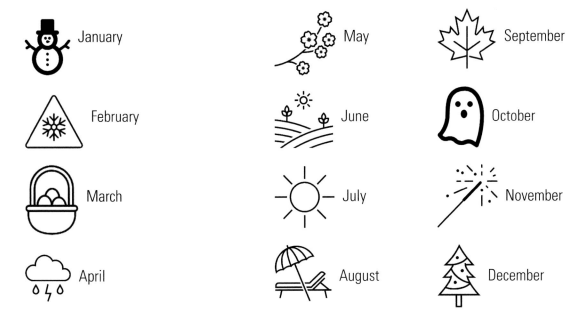

January

May

September

February

June

October

March

July

November

April

August

December

There are <u>12</u> months in a year and <u>4</u> seasons, each has <u>3</u> months

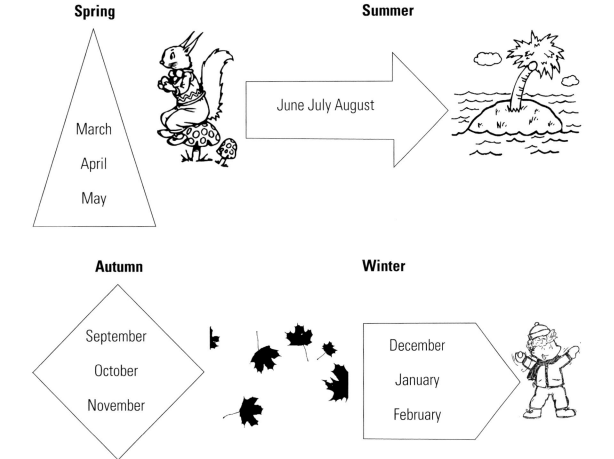

Spring

March
April
May

Summer

June July August

Autumn

September
October
November

Winter

December
January
February

The month before March is ....

The month before June is ....

The month after November is ....

The month after June is ....

The month after February is ....

The month before August is ....

The month before April is ....

Which season do the leaves fall? ....

Today the month is ....

How many seasons in a year?

Which season do we go to the beach?

Which season do we see baby chicks?

Two months in spring are ....

Two months in winter are ....

Is this right?

June and July are in the spring

October and September are in the summer

December and January are in the winter

July and August are in the winter

March is in the spring

August is in the summer

Useful words

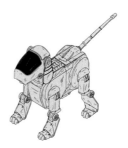

Multiply: Counting in groups of numbers.

Partition: Breaking a number into hundreds, ten and ones.

Addition (+): Words that mean the same, like Add, More, Plus, Total, Sum, Altogether.

Subtraction (−): Words that mean the same, like Take away, Minus, Less, what is the difference?

Grouping: Another word for multiplication.

Multiplication (x): Words that mean the same: Groups of, Product, Times.

Ordinal numbers: A number that tells you the position of something.

                                                     1st   2nd   3rd

Skip counting: It is similar to counting but missing numbers out.

2 4 6	5 10 15	10 20 30
in 2s	in 5s	in 10s

Fractions: They are a part of something.

1 A whole apple 1

2 A half an apple $\frac{1}{2}$

Key Stage 2 - Maths

Numbers

Remember the number tens and ones?

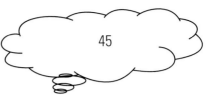

Numbers are made of digits. Digits are just another name for numbers.

0 1 2 3 4 5 6 7 8 9

Tens	Ones
4	5

We have learnt about tens and ones. Think about   98

It's made up of 9 tens and 8 ones

Now for the hundreds: The number **325**   This number is made up of 3 hundreds, 2 tens and 5 ones

The number **783**   This number is made up of 7 hundreds, 8 tens and 3 ones

Hundreds (H)	Tens (T)	Ones (O)
3	2	5
7	8	3

Can you please put these numbers in the correct boxes?

238   430   43   398   798   56   898   986   85

Hundreds	Tens	Ones

Remember skip counting?

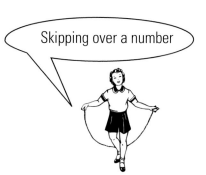

Skipping over a number

In **2s**

0 2 4 6 8 10 12 14 16 18 20 22 24 26
28 30 32 34 36 38 40 42 44 46 48 50

In **5s**

0   5   10   15   20   25   30   35   40   45   50

In **10s**

0   10   20   30   40   50

Counting in 10s from 16

1₆   2₆   3₆   4₆   5₆   6₆   7₆   8₆   9₆   10₆

The tens (number on the left) get bigger by one and the 6 in the ones (number on the right) column stays the same

Just increase the tens (number on the left) by one and leave the ones column alone

Can you count in 10s from 28 to 98?

Now for counting in hundreds – 100s

Not as hard as it sounds!

Counting in hundreds from 145

Think I do

You keep the tens and ones the same and make the hundreds bigger

1₄₅   2₄₅   3₄₅   4₄₅   5₄₅   6₄₅   7₄₅   8₄₅   9₄₅

Can you count from 120 to 920?

We learned about putting numbers in order with tens and ones

Put numbers with smallest tens first

55	33	21	89	78
21	33	55	78	89

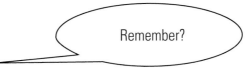

Remember?

These numbers have the same tens, but the ones are different. This time you look at the ones

54	50	51	58	59
50	51	54	58	59

Can you put these numbers in the right order?

67   88   82   12   65   17   19

Now for numbers with hundreds, tens, and ones

320   645   382   647

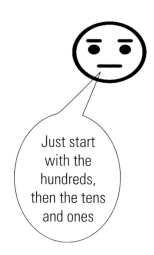

Just start with the hundreds, then the tens and ones

Hundreds	Tens	Ones
3	2	0
3	8	2
6	4	5
6	4	7

Can you put these numbers in order from smallest to biggest?

801   334   821   378   872   032

Another method is to use partitioning – looking at the hundreds, tens and ones in a different way

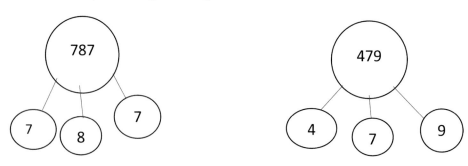

7 is the hundreds   8 is the tens   7 is the ones   4 is the hundreds   7 is the tens   9 is the ones

Can you partition these numbers this way?

783   332   769   440   450   119   117

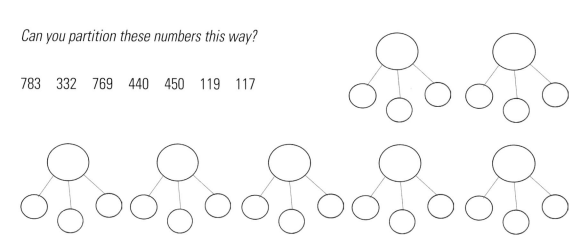

Adding again

Adding up with hundreds, tens and ones

We have learnt how to add before

```
  24          33
+ 12        + 25
────        ────
  36          58
────        ────
```

Easy – now a little tricky with ones that are bigger than 10

```
    T  O
+   2  7        Ones   7 + 5 = 12    1 ten and 2 ones    the ones go in the ones column as they
    2  5                                                 add up to more than 10
    (+1)                                                 the 1 ten is 'carried' (added) into the tens column
5      2
```

Here's another one

```
    T  O
+   3  6        6 + 9 = 15    1 ten and 5 ones    the ones go in the ones column,
    2  9                                          1 ten is 'carried' (added) into the tens column
    (+1)
6      5
```

Can you try these sums?

```
  T  O          T  O          T  O          T  O
+ 4  7        + 8  7        + 2  9        + 5  7
  2  4          1  9          6  5          4  8
  ____          ____          ____          ____
```

Now let's try adding with hundreds

```
  H  T  O
+ 5  6  4        4 + 2 = 6   ones  no need to carry − no tens
  2  7  2        6 + 7 = 13  tens   the  3 goes in the tens column and
  _____
  8  3  6        5 + 2 + 1 = 8   the 10 is carried into the hundreds column
 (+1)
```

Here's another one

```
  H   T  O
+ 6   8  8       8 + 6 = 14   The 4 ones go into the ones columns
  3   4  6       The 10 is carried (added) to the tens column  8 + 4 + 1 = 13
  _____
  10  3  4       The 3 goes into the tens column and the 1 added to the hundreds column
 (+1) (+1)
```

Here's some to try

```
  H  T  O          H  T  O          H  T  O          H  T  O
  2  7  8          5  7  3          2  6  9          2  8  9
+ 5  7  7        + 3  6  8        + 5  6  6        + 8  4  5
  _____        _____        _____        _____
```

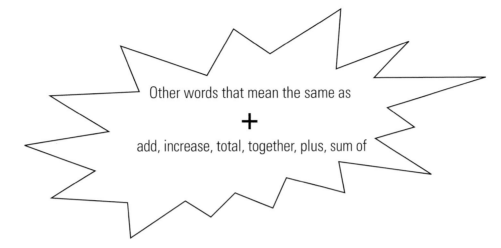

Other words that mean the same as

+

add, increase, total, together, plus, sum of

Some problems

Eric played 38 games this season and his friend Helena played 76. How many games did they play together?

Josh played 44 games for his team, the Solihull tigers and his friend Tiran played 49 for the same team. How many games did they play in total?

Joanna wants to make a fruit salad for the party. She buys 14 bananas, 25 apples and 32 oranges. Her friend Sadie buys 26 peaches and 1 pineapple. How many pieces of fruit did they buy altogether?

The library monitors, Jessica and Matthew, have to count up the books on History. They are on shelves. There are 235 on shelf 1, 322 on shelf 2 and 172 on shelf 3. How many books in total?

Subtraction again

It is a posh name for **take away**.   These ones are easy

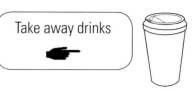

Take away drinks

```
T  0        Take away ones first   9 – 4

6  9        Then the tens  6 – 3

– 3  4
_____
3  5
```

Try these

```
T  0          T  0          T  0          T  0

8  7          5  9          5  7          8  6

– 4  3        – 3  7        – 3  6        – 5  3
_____        _____        _____        _____
```

It's easy because the numbers at the top are bigger

BUT   What happens when the ones on top are smaller?

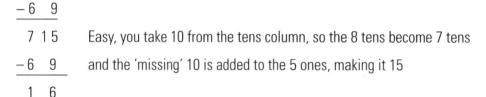

```
T  0

8  5        You can't take 9 away from 5.   Help, what can I do?

– 6  9
_____
7 1 5       Easy, you take 10 from the tens column, so the 8 tens become 7 tens

– 6  9      and the 'missing' 10 is added to the 5 ones, making it 15
_____
1  6
```

Another one

```
T    0       You can't take 9 away from 2.

5    12      So we take 10 from the tens column, so the 6 becomes 5

– 3   9      The 'missing' 10 is added to the 2 ones, it becomes 12
_____
2    3
```

See how you go with these:

```
  T   O        T   O        T   O        T   O
  7   4        8   2        4   2        9   1
- 3   7      - 5   8      - 1   9      - 6   9
_____      _____      _____      _____
```

Now let's try the hundreds

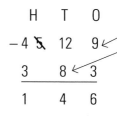

```
  H    T    O
- 4  ⁵1̶2    9
_____
  3    8    3
_____
  1    4    6
```

Let's look at the ones column. You can take 3 away from 9 no problem

Now the tens, you can't take 8 from 2 so you need to ask the 10s thief to help. He will take a 10 from the hundreds making the 2 into 12

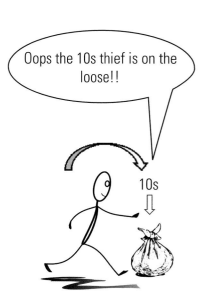

Oops the 10s thief is on the loose!!

10s

Another one

```
  H       T      O
  6̶7̶    ̶1̶1 0   (1)3
- 5       8       7
_____
  1       2       6
```

In the ones column you can't take 7 from 3 so we have to get help from the 10s thief and 3 becomes 13. 7 from 13 is 6

Because we borrowed from the tens there's 0 left so need to ask the 10s thief to take from the hundreds and as we now have a ten, 8 from 10 is 2

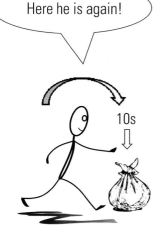

Here he is again!

10s

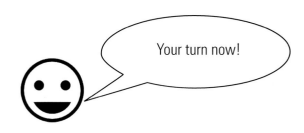

Your turn now!

H	T	O		H	T	O		H	T	O		H	T	O
4	8	6		3	6	2		8	1	4		6	1	8
−2	9	8		− 1	7	9		− 3	9	8		− 4	9	5

Other words that mean the same as subtraction

——

minus, take away, subtract, difference, fewer, deduct, how many left

Some subtraction problems

St. Marks Primary wants to raise £268 for the local hospital. So far they have raised £108. How much more do they need to reach their target?

Mat's flower shop made up 56 bunches of flowers. He sold 39. How many are left?

The Roxy cinema is showing Star Wars III. There are 437 seats in the cinema, 329 tickets have been sold. How many seats are left?

Ms. Stevens took in all year 4's books to mark. Altogether there are 127. So far she has marked 98. How many books has she left to mark?

Can you remember how to ......?

Count in 2s   0 2 4 6 8 10...48

Count in 5s   0 5 10 15 20 25...65

Count in 10s   0 10 20 30 40..120

Multiplication

Something new … Multiplication means 'times', 'lots of'.

Salim and Musta made 12 bags of sweets for the school fair.

Each bag had 8 sweets. If you want to find out how many sweets they have altogether:

You could just add $8 + 8 + 8 + 8 + 8 + 8 + 8 + 8 + 8 + 8 + 8 + 8$

But that takes forever!!

There's an easier way to find out …

The posh word for 'times' and 'lots of' is

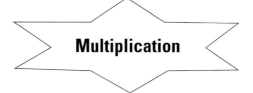

Multiplication

Jennifer has 4 baby dinosaurs and she feeds them 10 mice a day.

How many 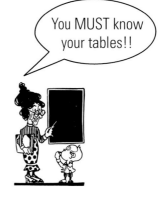 mice does she need to have every day?

As she has 4 baby dinosaurs, she needs $10 + 10 + 10 + 10 = 40$ mice

An easier way to find out would be to use **multiplication**

We have 4 lots of 10 in other words $4 \times 10 = 40$

Multiplication by one number, it's not unlike adding – **remember the rules!**

You MUST know your tables!!

```
T   0
5   5
 ×  5
─────
   275

+ 2
```

$5 \times 5 = 25$

The 5 goes in the ones column

The 2 is carried over to the tens column

5×5 is 25 plus the 2 carried over $25 + 2 = 27$

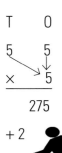

Try these:

```
    T   O        T   O
    6   4        7   8
×       4    ×       6
_____
```

Now with using Hundreds

```
    H   T   O    First: 4 × 4 = 16 put 6 in the ones  column
    2   1   4    Next: 4 × 1 = 4 + 1 carried over from ones column
×           4    Finally: 4 × 2 = 8 nothing to carry over to the hundreds column
_____
    8   5   6
       +1
```

Another one

```
    H   T   O    First:  5 × 4 = 20  0 goes in the ones column (O)  2 carried into tens column (T)
    9   3   4    Next:  5 × 3 = 15 + 2 carried into the T column the total is 17
×           5    Put 7 in tens column and 1 carried into the hundreds column (H)
_____
   46   7   0    Finally:  5 × 9 = 45 + 1 carried into the H column
  + 1  +2
```

Some to try:

```
    H   T   O        H   T   O        H   T   O        H   T   O
    6   7   8        5   6   9        3   8   7        8   5   4
×           5    ×           3    ×           4    ×           2
_____     _____     _____     _____
```

Multiplication problems

1. The stickers for football teams cost 30p for each packet. Jason wants to buy 3 of these, how much will it cost?

2. Joanne wants to buy new hair bands. Each band costs 15p each. How much will 5 of these cost?

3. Pat and Ralph were asked to put out 10 rows of chairs with 25 chairs in each row. How many chairs did they put out altogether?

4. There are 5 crates, each crate has 24 bottles of milk. How many bottles are there altogether?

5. In Class 4A there are 5 bookshelves. Each bookshelf has 34 books. How many books does the class have altogether?

Another look at multiplication

This time it's a little trickier – we have 2 digits! But don't worry! It's not that different from what we have learnt.

```
  5 1 6
×2 5
```

First step: let's look at it digit by digit, take the ones first

```
    516
×     5
  2580
```

Next step: multiply by tens, there are 2 tens

(Remember to put a 0 in the ones column as we are × by tens)

```
    516
×    20
10320
```

Last of all, we add both together

```
   2580
+10320
 12900
```

To Try:

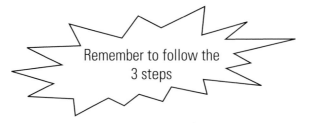

	H	T	O
		5	2
×		1	5

	H	T	O
		3	7
×		2	3

	H	T	O
		4	4
×		2	1

	H	T	O
		5	3
×		4	7

Remember to follow the 3 steps

1) First the ones   2) Then the tens   3) Add together

Here's an easy one before we leave multiplication for a while:

To multiply (make bigger) by 10 you add a 0 that's all!

Doubling of numbers

Earlier we learned how to double using addition of single numbers and tens

Doubling ones $6 + 6 = 12$ Doubling tens $20 + 20 = 40$

Now we will do 2- and 3-digit numbers by splitting them into tens and ones.

	T	O
	6	8
120	16

Double 6 tens is 120   Double 8 is 16

Add together $120 + 16 = 136$.

Another example

	T	O
	5	7
100	14

Double 5 tens is 100   Double 7 is 14

Add together $100 + 14 = 114$.

Can you double these numbers?

68   38   73   100   75   49   65

Some problems

Kerry bought a packet of biscuits for the party. There were only 24 in the packet, but she needs double that amount. How many biscuits does she need altogether?

Jack earns 80p for 1 hour helping in his garden. He helps for 2 hours, how much will he earn?

Doubling of 3 digits   HTO

$$320$$
$$600 + 40 = 640$$

$$430$$
$$800 + 60 = 860$$

Try at doubling these numbers

950   434   280   530   966   372   941   856   848   633   398

Remember when doubling 3 digits the hundreds column first then the tens and ones together

Mrs. Johnson has marked 110 exam papers but that's only half of them.
How many has she got to mark in total?

Kerrie has made 32 hot dogs for the school fair but she has to make the same number again.
How many must she make in total?

Division

When you share, everyone must have the same.

There are 6 pieces of pizza. Matt and Carly would like the same number of pieces each.

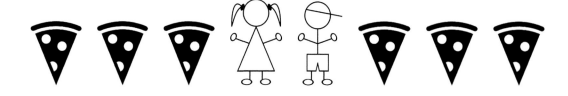

They have 3 pieces each, they have shared the pizza so they both have the same number. Another word for same is **equal**.

An easy way to share is to start off with giving them one each until there are none left.

Basil, Milo and Tigger are waiting for their fish. There are 9 pieces of fish. How many will each one get so they have equal numbers?

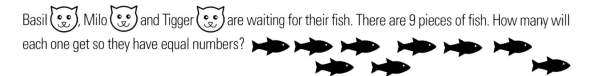

Another word for sharing is **dividing** but it means the same thing. It means it's quicker than doing 'one for you, one for me'.

James is feeding his 4 dogs; he is treating them to chicken. He has 8 pieces of chicken and needs to share them equally, or they will not be happy.

So we write $8 \div 4$ using the dividing sign. How many 4s are there in 8?

The answer is 2.

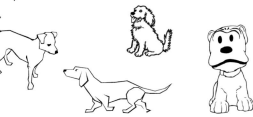

Each dog gets 2 pieces of chicken each

Using the division $\div$ sign

An easy one to start with

Share the lollipops between 4 people, 4 lollipops shared between 4 people $4 \div 4 = 1$

They get 1 each

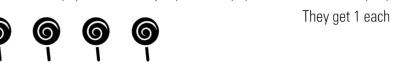

 10 ice creams $\div$ **5** children.   How many do they get each?

Try these

$$14 \div 7 =$$ $$12 \div 3 =$$ $$15 \div 5 =$$

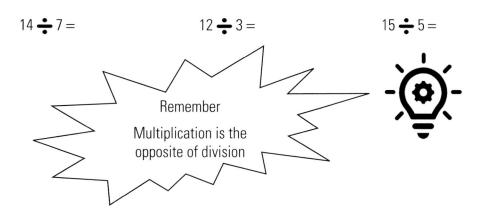

Remember

Multiplication is the opposite of division

Look at these examples:

$5 \times 3 = 15$ and $15 \div 3 = 5$

$6 \times 2 = 12$ and $12 \div 2 = 6$

$5 \times 3 = 15$ and $15 \div 3 = 15$

$2 \times 10 = 20$ and $20 \div 2 = 10$

$5 \times 5 = 25$ and $25 \div 5 = 5$

Can you put in the missing sign X or ÷ (multiplication or division)?

8 ? 2 = 16

6 ? 4 = 24

7 ? 5 = 35

10 ? 9 = 90

Can you put a missing sign in these sums and work out the answer?

16 ? 2 =

24 ? 4 =

35 ? 5 =

90 ? 10 =

Rounding off numbers

It means making the digits go up changing them to the nearest 5 or 10 it goes you a rough idea of an answer but not one that is really accurate.

If we use a number line, this helps to understand the idea

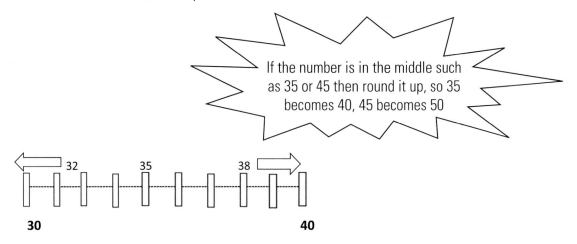

If the number is in the middle such as 35 or 45 then round it up, so 35 becomes 40, 45 becomes 50

If the **ones** of the number is **less** than 5, the number needs to be rounded **down**

If the **ones** of the number is 5 or **more**, the number needs to be rounded **up**

These rounded up and rounded down rules are the same for 100. This time looking at the **tens**

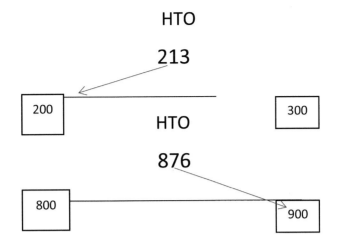

Try rounding these numbers to the nearest tens:

47…. 52…. 33…… 77…… 61… 82… 57…….

Try rounding these numbers to the nearest hundreds:

332 …… 207……. 689…… 463…… 1451….. 2503……

Can you remember? Multiplication by one digit

```
  H  T  O          H  T  O          H  T  O
  6  5  2          8  8  9          5  8  7
×        4        ×        3        ×        4
_____         _____         _____
```

Some subtraction sums:

```
  H  T  O          H  T  O          H  T  O          H  T  O
  4  6  8          8  6  7          6  4  7          8  9  4
− 2  4  8          1  7  9          4  9  8          3  7  8
_____         _____         _____         _____
```

Fractions

Don't worry, it's bit like sharing

Here's a pizza, Matt and Chris **love** pizza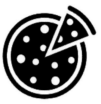

Mum has bought 1 whole pizza and makes sure they both have equal pieces, so she cuts it in half.
You write half like this $\frac{1}{2}$

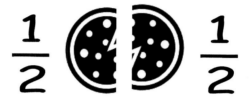

2 halves make 1 whole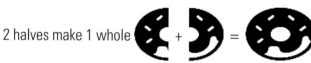

$$\frac{1}{2} + \frac{1}{2} = 1 \text{ whole}$$

Can you colour in half of these apples?

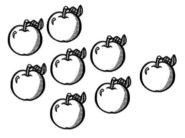

How many have you coloured in? Half of 8 is ?

There are 10 cakes, draw a circle round half of them. What is half of 10 ?

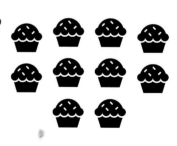

Colour $\frac{1}{2}$ of the rabbit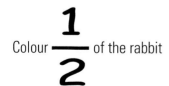

Shapes

So far, we have learnt some shapes

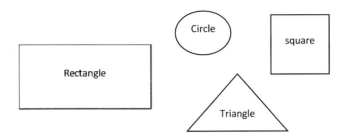

Here are some new ones to learn. These are not really too different. The rhombus is like a square pushed over and the parallelogram like a rectangle pushed over.

These are all flat shapes – they are called **2D shapes**.

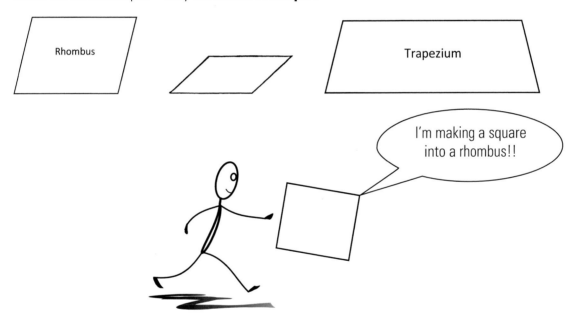

3D shapes

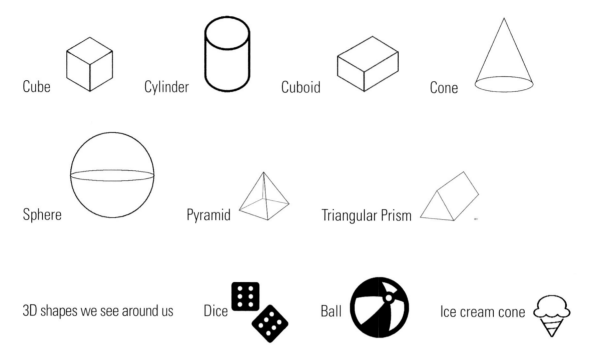

Cube   Cylinder   Cuboid   Cone

Sphere   Pyramid   Triangular Prism

3D shapes we see around us   Dice   Ball   Ice cream cone

Can you think of any more 3D shapes we see all around us?

Here are some words that describe 3D shapes and you have to learn them:

It's a corner, but you have to call it a **Vertex**
(Vertices: more than one)

An easy one **Face**

Another easy one **Edge** (where the faces meet)

You have to know how to describe each shape. It makes it easier to recognise when you see it. Find an object in the classroom you can recognise by its shape.

So, it's not too bad!

Let's start with a cube. Find a dice or square brick

Cube

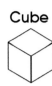

1st Count the **faces**   It has ……….faces

2nd Count the **edges**   It has ……..edges

3rd Count the **vertices** (corners)   It has …….vertices

A sphere (ball)

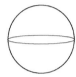

Does it have any edges?

Does it have any vertices?

How many faces does it have?

A cuboid (piece of Lego rectangle shape)

Cuboid

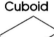

It has ……….edges   It has …. faces

It has ……vertices   Are the edges all the same length?

Which **3D** shape has   1 flat face, 1 vertex, no edges, 1 curved surface?

Which **3D** shape has   5 faces,   2 are triangular faces,   3 are rectangular faces?

Which **2D** shape has   4 straight lines all the same length and 4 corners?

Which **3D** shape has   2 flat and circular faces, 1 curved surface and no edges?

More fractions

So far, we have looked at dividing or sharing things in half such as pizza, doughnut, cake.

Now we 'll look at quarters

Jason, Sacha, Petra and Jack all want some pizza. There are 4 of them, so it has to be divided into quarters.

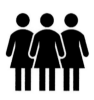 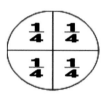 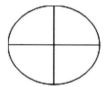

Can you shade in two *halves of this circle?*

Two are the same as ....?

How much of the circle is **not** shaded?

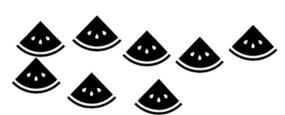

Tracy has 4 friends coming to see her

They like watermelon so she has cut 8 pieces

They will each get $\frac{1}{4}$

How many will each one get?

Tracy has made an apple pie and has asked two of her friends to share it with her. Tracy has to make sure they have equal shares. There are three of them so each person will have one-third

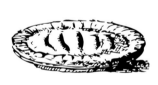 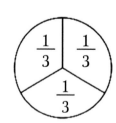

3 one-thirds = **1** whole

Can you shade in one-third of the shape?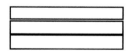

Time

We learned about knowing when we say 'o'- CLOCK when both the small and big hands are together

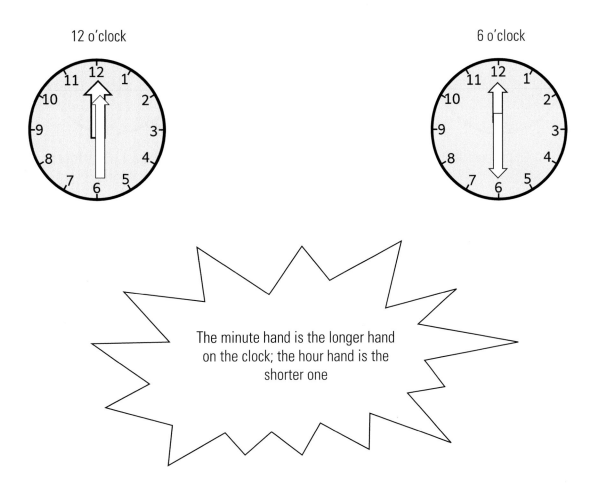

The minute hand is the longer hand on the clock; the hour hand is the shorter one

The clock is divided into 12 bits (sections), each one lasts 5 minutes so remember your counting in 5s?

It's very important to help you tell the time

Here's a reminder   0 5 10 15 20 25 30 35 40 45 50 55

Past the hour

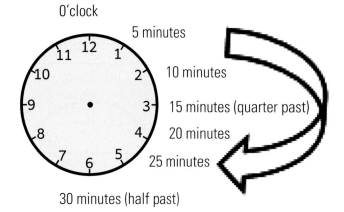

O'clock

5 minutes

10 minutes

15 minutes (quarter past)

20 minutes

25 minutes

30 minutes (half past)

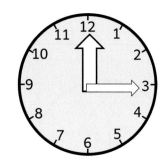

15 minutes past 12 (quarter past)

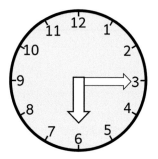

30 minutes past 3 (half past)

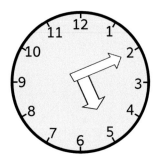

10 minutes past 5

Moving towards the next hour

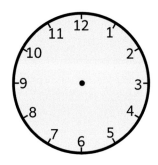

Can you draw 5 minutes past 4 on the clock?

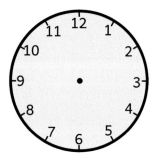

Can you draw 10 minutes past 8 on the clock?

Time problems

Jane started her swimming practice at 4 pm and swam for 1 hr 10 minutes. What time did she finish?

Paul began his football practice at 1 pm and stopped at 3.20 pm. How long was the football practice?

The rain started at 12.30 pm and finished at 2.00 pm. How long was it raining?

After half past you have to tell the time to the next hour. A little tricky!!

I must remember no more saying 'past' once the minute hand has moved after half past or 30 minutes. It's now going towards the next hour

Towards the next hour

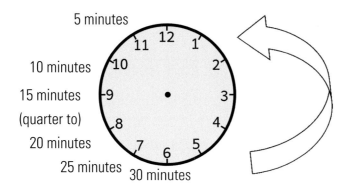

5 minutes

10 minutes

15 minutes
(quarter to)

20 minutes

25 minutes 30 minutes

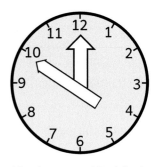

10 minutes to 12 o'clock

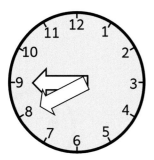

20 minutes to 9 o'clock

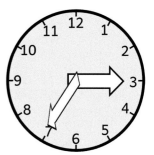

25 minutes to 3 o'clock

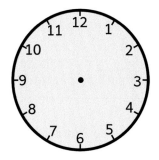

Can you draw a quarter to 11 on the clock?

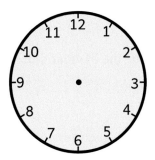

Can you draw 5 minutes to 4 on the clock?

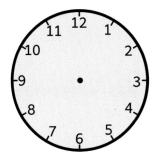

Can you draw 20 minutes past 5 on the clock?

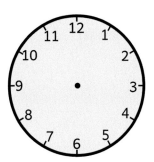

Can you draw half past 7 on the clock?

Time problems

Jason had to play tennis for 25 minutes and started at 25 minutes to 4. What time did he finish?

Stacey started dancing at 20 minutes to 6. What time did she finish?

The exercise class started at a quarter to 7 and lasted for 1 hour 15 minutes. What time did it finish?

Digital and the 24-hour clock

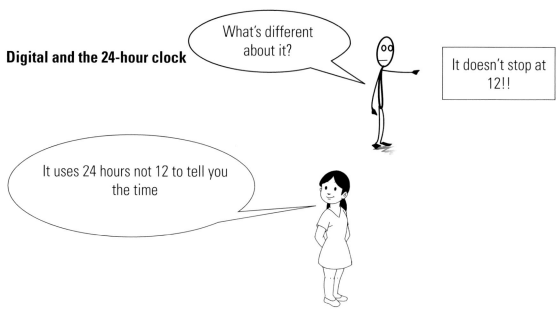

What's different about it?

It doesn't stop at 12!!

It uses 24 hours not 12 to tell you the time

Always remember

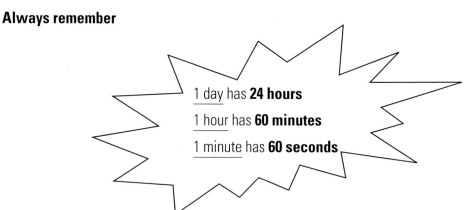

1 day has **24 hours**

1 hour has **60 minutes**

1 minute has **60 seconds**

Here's some more examples: The clock says 20 minutes past 11 o'clock. We don't know if it is morning or evening

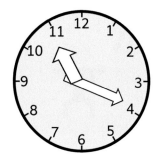

It looks the same, if we mean morning or evening.

If we mean the morning, we write it 11.20 **am**

If we mean the evening, we write it 11.20 **pm**

The only difference is **am** or **pm**, so it tells you: morning or evening

With the 24-hour clock, you add (+) 12 to show you mean after midday so 11.20 pm = 23:20

If its 11.20 am, it looks almost the same = 11:20. For times before 10.00 am you add a 0

08:00 = 8 am   20.00 = 8 pm   05:00 = 5.00 am   17:00 = 5 pm

9.00 pm = 21:00   digital   6.15 pm = 18:15   6.15 am = 06:15

2.30 pm = 14:30   digital   3.45 pm = 15:45   3.45 am = 03:45

3.15 am = 03:15   digital   8.30 pm = 20:30   8.30 am = 08:30

Midnight, my favourite time is 00:00
just before it is 23:59

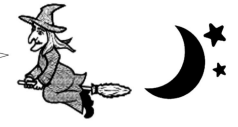

*Can you put these digital clock times
into am or pm?*

07:20 =   10:00 =

13: 45 =   18:30 =

21:20 =   05:00 =

17:30 =   23:25 =

23:59 =   00:00 =

*Can you put these am or pm clock times into
digital?*

7.15 am =   5.30 am =

8.20 pm =   6.50 pm =

6.10 pm =   9.15 pm =

3.45 am =   8.25 pm =

11 pm =   3.30 pm =

Some problems

1. Jack started running at 07:30. He ran for 25 minutes. What time did he stop?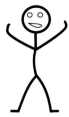

2. Jason went to the cinema. The film started at 17:30 and lasted 1 hour 30 minutes. What time did it finish?

3. Sean and Gaby started walking at 19:15. They walked for 30 minutes. What time did they finish?

4. Bethany started her homework at 18:05 and finished at 19:00. How long did it take her?

5. Johan and Beth decided to walk to the beach. They thought that it would take them 20 minutes. They started at 6.30 and arrived there at 7.00. Did it take longer than they thought? By how many more minutes?

6. Sita and Yasmin started to bake a cake at 5.15. They had finished it by 6.00. How long did it take them?

More money!

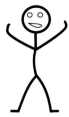   £ £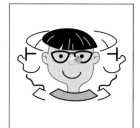

We have learnt about money

  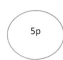 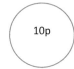

1p   2p   5p   10p   20p   50p

Adding:

10p + 20p = 30p   5p + 10p = 15p   20p + 50p = 70p

20p + 20p + 20p + 20p + 20p = £1   50p + 50p = £1

10 + 10 + 10 + 10 + 10 + 10 + 10 + 10 + 10p + 10p = £1

One
pound

£1

50p + 30p + 20p =

5p + 20p + 5p + 20p + 50p =

1p + 1p + 1p + 1p + 1p + 50p + 20p + 5p + 10p + 10p =

Draw 2 coins which make £1   Draw 5 coins which make £1   Draw 3 coins which make £1

Can you think of two different ways of making £1?

Adding up with money – not really different from ordinary adding up

        £9.57
    + £9.66
    ─────────
      £19.23p
        1 1

Try these

£ 3. 67	£ 9.68	£ 7.34
+ £ 9. 28	+ 4.37	+ 2.85

Multiplying money, it's the same

£ 5.30

×   5

──────

26 .50

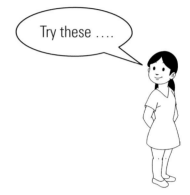

Try these ….

£6.92 + £2.82 =   £18.44 − £5.12 =

£3.24 × 3 =   £5.35 × 2 =

Money problems:

1. Simon ate 10 salt and mustard sandwiches. Each sandwich costs 55p. How much did they cost altogether?

2. Sacha wants Fortnite Lego, which costs £7.45. Betsy wants a disco mic, which costs £9.50. What is the total cost?

3. Janet had £8.50 to spend, she bought a new pen for £3.50 and 2 exercise books for £1.50 each. How much does she have left?

4. Jake spends £1.20 on two apples and an orange. The apples cost 45p each . How much did the banana cost?

5. Lucy and her brother James have £1 to spend, they would like a slice of pizza each . One slice costs 55p. Does she have enough money?

Remember division

Dividing when things get smaller.

We've done halving, dividing numbers like $12 \div 6$

Now we'll try division in a different way. It's called short division, but sometimes called the bus stop method because it looks a bit like a bus. It's different from the other sorts of sums as the answer is put on top.

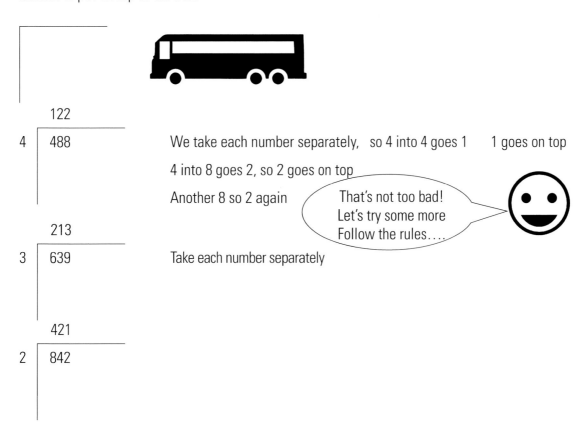

```
    122
4 | 488
```
We take each number separately, so 4 into 4 goes 1   1 goes on top

4 into 8 goes 2, so 2 goes on top

Another 8 so 2 again

That's not too bad! Let's try some more Follow the rules….

```
    213
3 | 639
```
Take each number separately

```
    421
2 | 842
```

Now just a little bit harder

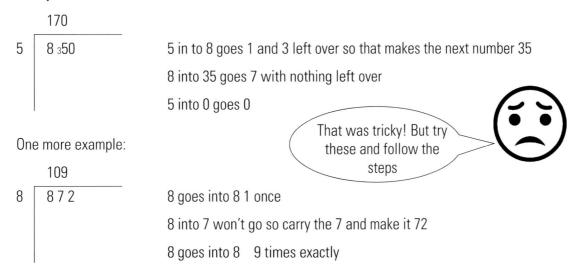

```
    170
5 | 8 ₃50
```
5 in to 8 goes 1 and 3 left over so that makes the next number 35

8 into 35 goes 7 with nothing left over

5 into 0 goes 0

That was tricky! But try these and follow the steps

One more example:

```
    109
8 | 8 7 2
```
8 goes into 8 1 once

8 into 7 won't go so carry the 7 and make it 72

8 goes into 8   9 times exactly

6 | 6 3 6   7 | 7 4 9   5 | 535

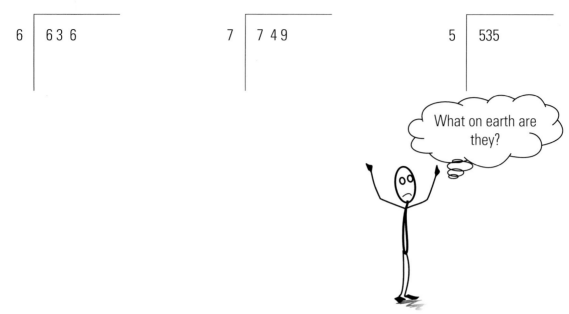

Decimals: the in-between numbers

They're useful to tell you that a number is in between two numbers. We've done rounding off when, if a number is, say, 57 we'd round it off to 60. It's a bit like rounding off but to have a better idea of where the number really is, you use a dot. it's called a **decimal point**. To see how we would put the numbers 5.3, 5.7 and 5.9 in order:

Tens		Ones	(not quite tens)
5	.	3	It's just a bit bigger than 5 but not much
5	.	7	Bigger than 5.3 but not as big as
5	.	9	It's almost 6! .

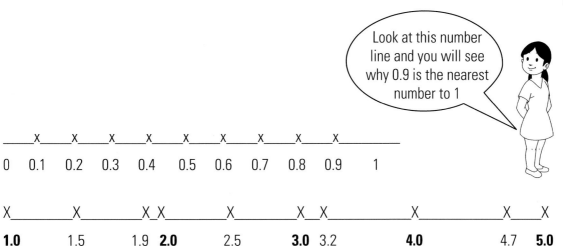

Look at this number line and you will see why 0.9 is the nearest number to 1

```
____X____X____X____X____X____X____X____X____X_____
0   0.1  0.2  0.3  0.4  0.5  0.6  0.7  0.8  0.9   1
```

```
X_____X_____X_X_____X_____X__X_____X_____X____X
1.0       1.5      1.9 2.0    2.5      3.0 3.2     4.0        4.7  5.0
```

Which is the number nearest to 2.0?   Is 3.2 bigger or smaller than 3.0?

Can you put these numbers in the right order from smallest to largest?

0.4   0.2   0.1 0.6 0.8 1   2.1   2.6   2.7 3.0   3.3 3.1 3.7 4.0

Now we'll try 2 decimal places – which one is nearest to 3.0?   2.80 is nearer to 3 than 2.10

```
X_____X_____X_____X_____X_____X_____X_____X_____X_____X_____X_
2.0    2.10   2.20   2.30   2.40   2.50   2.60   2.70   2.80   2.90   3.00
```

Can you put these numbers in order from biggest to smallest?

0.4   1.02 3.09   0.01   3.08   5.02

Adding and subtracting with decimals

Don't worry they're no different but remember to line up those decimal points

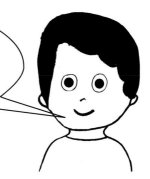

```
  5. 4        3. 52       4 ⁵1 2       5 ⁶1 3
 +2. 5       + 2. 35      –   2.8      – 4.  9
 ─────       ───────      ───────      ───────
  7.9          5.87        2 .4         1.  4
```

Remember you can't take 8 away from 2 so you need this chap again!

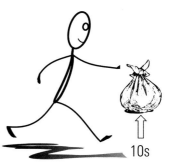

10s

Multiplying and dividing with ordinary numbers and decimals

As we've seen before, to multiply by 10 you add a zero, so $35 \times 10 = 350$

To multiply by 100 you add 2 zeros, so $35 \times 100 = 3500$

To multiply by 1000, it's 3 zeros $35 \times 1000 = 35000$ *Eeeesy peeesy!*

It's easy to multiply numbers like 20, 400, etc.

$231 \times 300 =$ First step $231 \times 3 = 693$ then add the 2 zeros to add the hundreds 69300

Can you do these:

$568 \times 10 =$	$305 \times 200 =$	$423 \times 300 =$	$511 \times 100 =$
$610 \times 10 =$	$723 \times 2000 =$	$601 \times 2000 =$	$525 \times 30 =$

Now we come to multiplying numbers with a decimal point.

We can't just add zeros it wouldn't make the number any bigger. Look at 3.50×10, if you add another 0 it becomes 3.500 and the number isn't any bigger. You've just put a zero which means nothing.

We know that multiplying makes the number bigger, move the decimal point to the right:
$3.50 \times 10 = 35.0$ (you add a ??? $\boxed{}\!\!\!\Longrightarrow$ Zero if necessary)

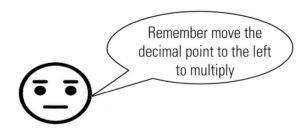

Remember move the decimal point to the left to multiply

$3.70 \times 10 = 37.0$

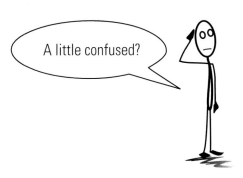

A little confused?

$46.25 \times 10 = 462.5$

$8.45 \times 10 = 84.5$

Try these $43.25 \times 10 =$ $35.35 \times 10 =$ $55.35 \times 10 =$ $8.55 \times 10 =$ $165.25 \times 10 =$

Move the point to the right to make the number **bigger** $\times$ **10** $\Longrightarrow$ **1** place

$\times$ **100** $\Longrightarrow$ **2** places

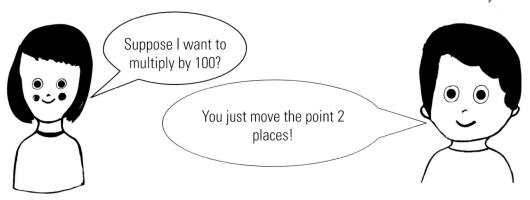

Suppose I want to multiply by 100?

You just move the point 2 places!

$428 \times 100 = 42800$ $33.78 \times 100 = 3378$ $208.00 \times 100 = 20800$

$245.617 \times 100 = 24561.7$ $54.8 \times 100 = 5480$ $77.8 \times 100 = 7780$

Try these: $254.312 \times 100 =$ $33.9 \times 100 =$ $78.6 \times 100 =$ $309 \times 100 =$ $76.6 \times 10 =$

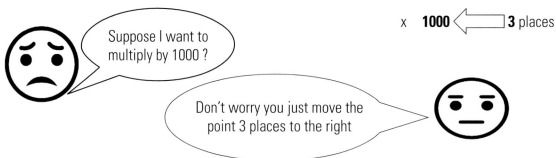

x **1000** ⟵ **3** places

Suppose I want to multiply by 1000 ?

Don't worry you just move the point 3 places to the right

$456 \times 1000 = 456000$ $64.88 \times 1000 = 64880$ $37.97 \times 1000 = 37970$

$9.7853 \times 1000 = 9785.3$ $8.476 \times 1000 = 8.476.0$ $309.34 \times 100 =$ $7469 \times 100 =$

Remember, we have learnt about dividing using the bus stop method and also in a line

$8 \div 2 = 4$ $24 \div 2 = 12$

Sharing or dividing makes the number smaller

If there are zeros at the end and you want to divide by 10 you just knock off the 0

$200 \div 10 = 20$ $460 \div 10 = 46$ $45000 \div 10 = 4500$

Can you try these? $500 \div 10 =$ $4700 \div 100 =$ $45 \times 100 =$ $33 \times 1000 =$ $6 \times 10 =$

What do you think we do with decimal numbers?

Umm ....do we move the point the other way?

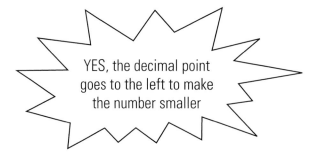

YES, the decimal point goes to the left to make the number smaller

$164 \div 10 = 16.4$ There are no zeros so we move a decimal point one place to the left to ÷ by

10 ⟹ 1 place

Try these:

$800 \div 10 =$ $19.8 \div 10 =$ $240 \div 10 =$ $45.6 \div 10 =$ $3400 \div 10 =$

You don't need to put a zero at the end of a number, so $2400 \div 100$ is written as 24.

To divide by 100, remember we're making the number smaller. How many places do we move that decimal point? And which way?

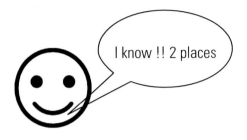

I know !! 2 places

I know this as well ! It's to the right

$694 \div 100 = 6.94$ $3400 \div 100 = 34$ $2413 \div 100 = 24.13$ $66.5 \div 100 = 0.665$

$4.6 \div 100 = 0.046$ $2.0 \div 100 = 0.020 = 0.02$ You don't need the zero at the end

Try these:

$900 \div 100 =$ $6.7 \div 100 =$ $5.00 \div 100 =$

$78.9 \div 100 =$ $4500 \div 100 =$ $7.79 \div 100 =$ $8.0 \div 100 =$

Why the zero?

You have to put in a zero or two in case you run out of numbers

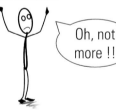

Oh, not more !!

Almost there but we're now looking at dividing numbers by 1000

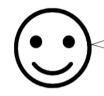

That means
3 zeros or moving
the decimal point
3 places

$189000 \div 1000 = 189$ $196820 \div 1000 = 196.82$

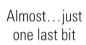

Remember the zero because
you've probably run out of digits

$625 \div 1000 = 0.625$ $56.90 \div 1000 = 0.056.9$ $91.67 \div 1000 = 0.091.67$

$5000 \div 1000 = 5$ $700 \div 1000 = 0.7$ $203 \div 1000 = 0.203$

Try these:

$755 \div 1000 =$ $88.90 \div 1000 =$ $7000 \div 1000 =$ $60.4 \div 1000 =$

$20 \div 1000 =$ $20.5 \div 100 =$ $750 \div 100 =$

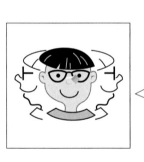

Phew my head's
spinning!! Have we
finished?

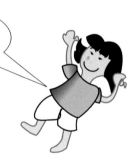

Almost…just
one last bit

A few problems…

1. Jen gets £0.10p for collecting bottles. How much will she get if she collects 100 bottles?
2. 1000 children in the school collect 20p each. How much will they have collected altogether?
3. Altogether there are 300 pencils to give out to 10 pupils. How many pencils will each one get?
4. The disco has put out 200 drinks of lemonade. There are 100 pupils, how many drinks will each one get?

Multiplying with decimals

$0.6 \times 4 = ?$

Step 1.   Forget about the decimal so it's 6×4

Step 2.   What is the product (answer) of $6 \times 4 = 24$

Step 3.   Now for the decimal point. How many numbers after the decimal point in both numbers? In this case, one after the tens. Place the decimal point after the tens. The answer: 2.4

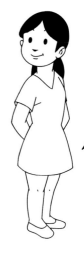

Just thought I'd show you how to multiply with decimals

$2.4\,3 \times 0.2 = ?$

Step 1.   Forget about the decimal, 243×2

Step 2.   243

$\quad\quad \times \quad 2$

$\quad\quad \overline{4\ 8\ 6}$

Step 3.   How many numbers **after** the decimal point for both the numbers? Start from the right, 3 places   Answer: 0.486

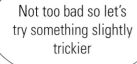

Not too bad so let's try something slightly trickier

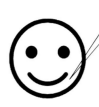

Here's a few to try:

$3.5 \times 0.2 =$ $\quad\quad\quad 2.3 \times 0.3 =$ $\quad\quad\quad 2.44 \times 0.2 =$ $\quad\quad\quad 3.6 \times 0.4 =$

$1.57 \times 0.3 =$ $\quad\quad\quad 4.2 \times 0.3 =$ $\quad\quad\quad 2.8\,8 \times 0.2 =$ $\quad\quad\quad 1.6\,6 \times 0.5 =$

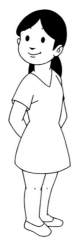

Columns and rows

Columns go downwards, while rows go across.

Columns go downwards

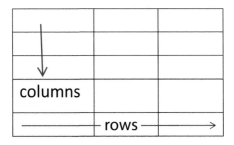

Rows go across

Useful words

2-D shapes: Flat like paper.

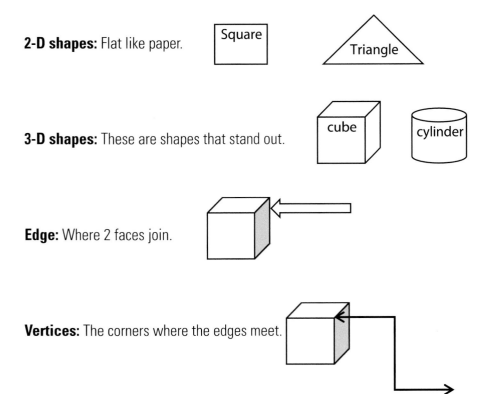

3-D shapes: These are shapes that stand out.

Edge: Where 2 faces join.

Vertices: The corners where the edges meet.

Digital clock: Uses 24 hours to tell the time.

Decimals: A way of writing a number that is not a whole one. They are 'in between numbers'. 10.3 is in between the numbers 10 and 11.

To make a decimal number bigger, you move the point to the right.   5.7 ➡ 57

To make a decimal number smaller, you move the point to the left.   14 ⬅ 1.4

Partitioning: A way of splitting numbers into hundreds, tens and ones.

Rounding off numbers: Moving numbers upwards or downwards to their nearest 10.
For example: 53 would be rounded down to 50,   57 is closer to 60. As a rule, if the last digit ends with 1,2,3,4, it is rounded down to the nearest 10. If the last digit is 5, 6,7,8,9, it is rounded up to the nearest 10.

Columns and rows: Columns go downwards, while rows go across.

Key Stage 1 - English

There are different parts of speech. We give names to different words which make up English. We'll start with nouns…

Nouns

A noun is a **naming** word. It can name a person, thing or place such as a nurse, a teacher, footballer, a cat, a dinosaur, a school, a house, a shop.

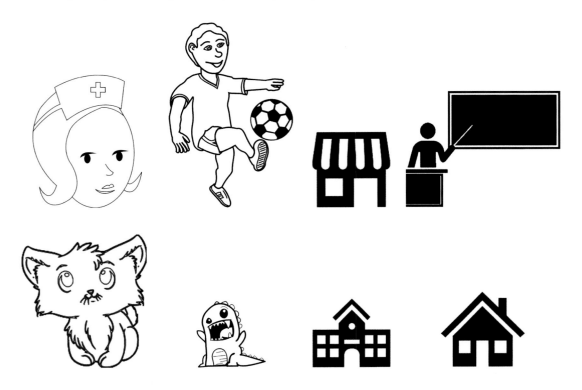

To help you find the noun in a sentence, you ask Who? or What?

The bird was pretty.   Who was pretty? **The bird**
The cake was tasty.   What was tasty? **The cake**
The leaves had fallen.   What had fallen? **The leaves**

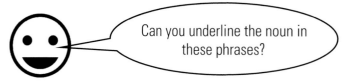

Can you underline the noun in these phrases?

The dog was noisy.   The lady jumped.   The T-shirt is too big.
The cat is pretty.   The car was comfortable.

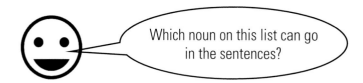

Which noun on this list can go in the sentences?

The .... flew above.

The .... was broken.

The .... was too small. | bear   plane   table   elephant |
                                    | cup   coat   bird |
The .... was huge.

The .... growled.

Circle the one which fits the description.

Which one lives in water?

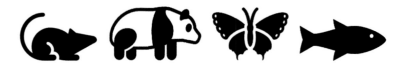

Which one helps you to write?

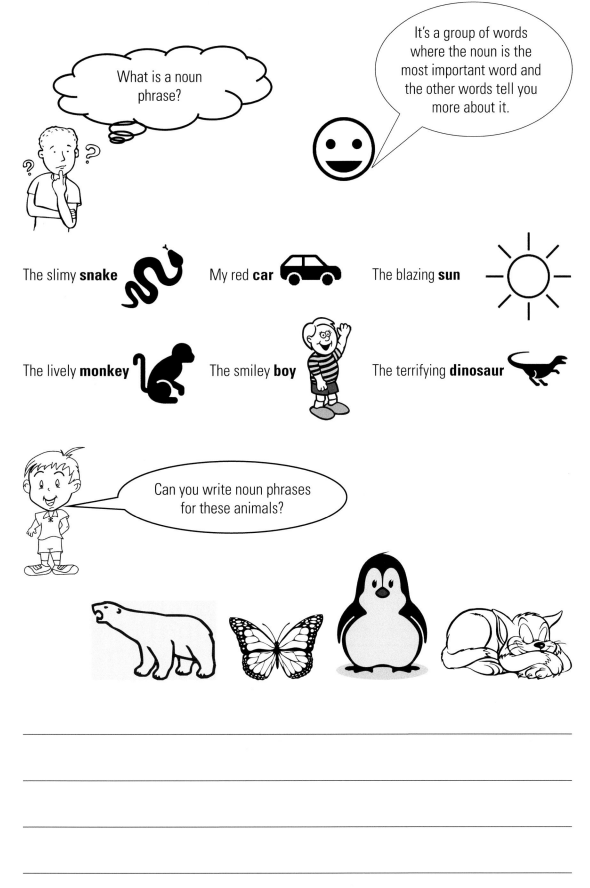

Verbs

Verbs can be part of a simple noun phrase, e.g.   My hand **is** warm.

Verbs tell you what someone or something is doing. To find the verb in a sentence, you ask the question, what or who is doing what?

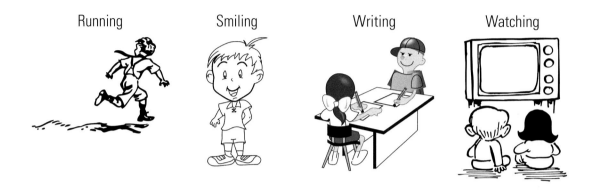

| Running | Smiling | Writing | Watching |

The boy is **running** down the road. What is the boy doing? He is **running**, the verb is **running**, which tells you what the boy is doing.

John is **smiling**. What is John doing? He is **smiling**.

Peter and Salina are **writing**. What are Peter and Salina doing? They are **writing**.

The children are **watching** the television. What are the children doing? They are **watching**.

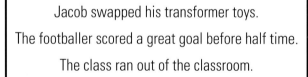

Jacob swapped his transformer toys.

The footballer scored a great goal before half time.

The class ran out of the classroom.

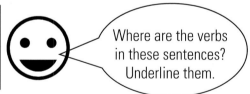

Where are the verbs in these sentences? Underline them.

There are two verbs in these sentences, can you find them?

The bright sun shone, and everyone went swimming.

The snow covered the houses and the children made a snowman.

The fox crept into the hen house and ate the chickens.

The rain beat down and James looked for his umbrella.

Adjectives

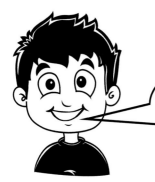

I know about nouns and verbs, but they are rather boring on their own. We need an **adjective** as it makes sentences more interesting.

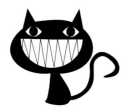

The **fierce** cat.   Fierce tells you more about the cat.

Fierce is an **adjective**

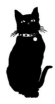

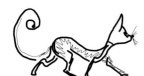

The **black** cat.   Black is an **adjective**

The **skinny** cat.   Skinny is an **adjective**

Adjectives give a helping hand to the nouns.

We found a mouse in our new house. Is sort of ok but…

We found a **cheeky** mouse in our new house is more interesting.

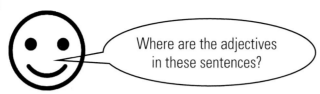

Where are the adjectives in these sentences?

The house was cold.

Brian had new shoes.

The beautiful butterfly flew over the grass.

The pretty girl went to a party.

There are two adjectives in these sentences, can you find them?

The grass was cold and damp.

The wind whistled through the damp, dark cave.

It was a freezing, cold morning.

Jane ruined her beautiful new dress.

Complete the sentences with an adjective from the ones in the boxes

delicious	slice	scary	fast

exciting	beautiful	difficult	large

Jane chose a .... pastry.

The princess wore a .... dress at the ball.

The ...... cake was enjoyed by all.

Jennifer is a very .... runner and she won easily.

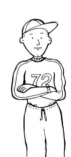

Jack found his homework very ....

Jonathan likes to watch .... football.

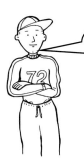

Can you now choose adjectives to describe this spooky house?

The children were frightened of the ... . house.

The ... . moon shone, and it looked so ....

old	small	creepy	clean

silvery	hung	slow	pale	ugly

Can you find two adjectives to describe Sid the snake?

Sid the snake is....... and ...

Helpful hint....
What colour could he be? Is he smooth or rough to touch?

What can you say about Sam the Shark?

Sam is a ......fish. He has ....teeth which he uses to eat up the little fishes.

Adverbs

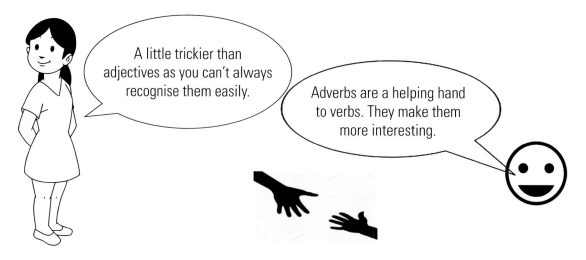

A little trickier than adjectives as you can't always recognise them easily.

Adverbs are a helping hand to verbs. They make them more interesting.

Jane laughed is ok, but Jane laughed **loudly** is better. We know how she laughed. **Loudly** is an adverb.

Peter ate his dinner quickly. **Quickly** tells you how he ate his dinner. **Quickly** is an adverb.

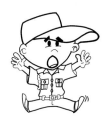

Phil screamed yesterday. **Yesterday** tells you when Phil screamed. **Yesterday** is an adverb.

Some adverbs tell you where something is happening.

The birds flew above. **Above** tells you where the birds flew. **Above** is an **adverb**.

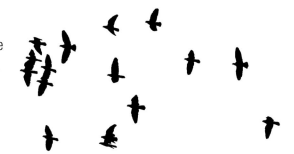

Can you find the adverbs in these sentences?

Peter walked cautiously down the road.

He had to walk to school quickly.

Carefully, Joanne wrapped the present.

We are going out tomorrow.

Jack, our cat will come home later.

Joanne danced happily down the street.

Can you make up a sentence for each of these three adverbs?

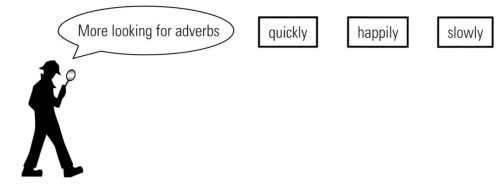

| quickly | happily | slowly |

Where is it happening?

The cat was curled up inside the cupboard.

The dog barked outside the house.

The mess was everywhere.

Can you make up three separate sentences with adverbs which tell you where things are happening?

| downstairs | below | around |

When did it happen?

I will come and see you tomorrow.

I saw my dad recently.

I never go out late.

Can you make sentences using these adverbs?

| later | always | earlier |

Remember: Adverbs do not always end in **ly**. They can also tell you where and when events happen.

Punctuation . ? ! ,

Capital letters and full stops

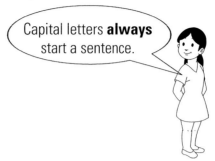

Capital letters **always** start a sentence.

The fox went into the chicken run.   **W**e are going to the zoo today.   **T**he apples are ready.

If you write:

we will go to see the film soon

It doesn't look right, no capital letter or full stop

It should be: We will go to see the film soon.

That's not all. You **must** put a full stop at the end of a sentence.

What about these, can you write them out accurately?

he said we can't come out.   it's easy to do the sums

the boys will come out later   the shops are closed today

you need more than 30p to buy the sweets

Which ones here have I remembered to use capital letters and full stops?

Bertie the cat walked away slowly.   Slowly the snake made his way across the forest

he will see you tomorrow.   afterwards we'll go to the cinema.

yesterday the weather was awful   he said we must be there at five o'clock

A FULL STOP tells you it's the end of a sentence. BUT this is not always what happens at the end of a sentence.

Question mark

When we ask a question, we use a question mark **?**

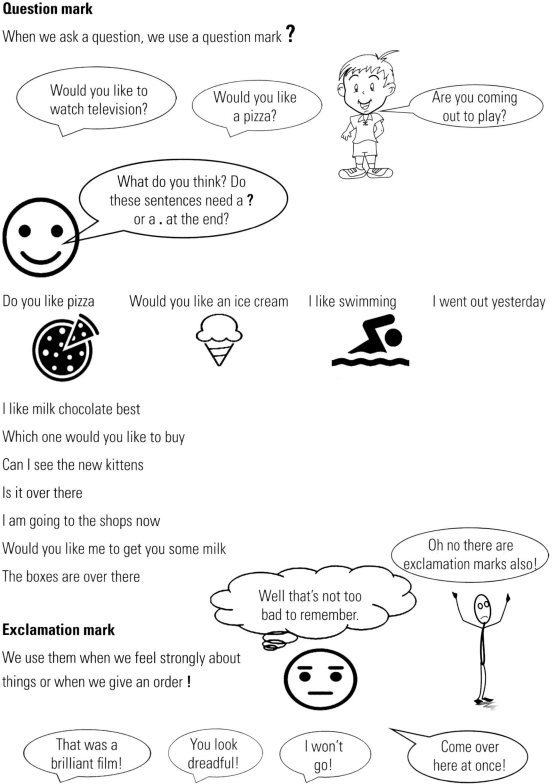

Would you like to watch television?

Would you like a pizza?

Are you coming out to play?

What do you think? Do these sentences need a **?** or a **.** at the end?

Do you like pizza

Would you like an ice cream

I like swimming

I went out yesterday

I like milk chocolate best

Which one would you like to buy

Can I see the new kittens

Is it over there

I am going to the shops now

Would you like me to get you some milk

The boxes are over there

Exclamation mark

We use them when we feel strongly about things or when we give an order **!**

Well that's not too bad to remember.

Oh no there are exclamation marks also!

That was a brilliant film!

You look dreadful!

I won't go!

Come over here at once!

Which sentences need an exclamation mark?

Come here now

I like going to the cinema

Can I have a drink please

Shall we go now

Are you ready

Stop it at once

I think you look very well

Go away now

Come on let's run fast

Stop talking at once

Wait for me

Be quick now

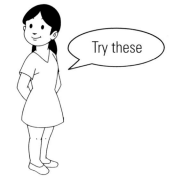

Try these

Can you put the right punctuation at the end of the sentences?

Is it time yet   The cartoon starts at 3 o'clock

Hurry up at once   I like your new transformers

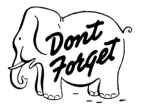

A capital letter always starts a sentence

Don't Forget

At the end of a sentence you can have . ! ?

We know about capital letters at the start of a sentence BUT … We can have capital letters at other times as well.

Whenever it's the specific name of a person, for example: The winner was Paul.

Capital letters

When we talk about a country – England, Scotland or a place London.

Days of the week – Monday, Tuesday, Wednesday, Thursday, Friday, Saturday, Sunday.

Months of the year – January, February, March, etc.

When you talk about yourself using **I,** you always use a capital letter as I is an important person. For example:

I went to the shops yesterday. I like fish and chips and I also like burger and chips.

Ben and I went to the gym on Thursday.

Which of these nouns need a capital letter?

friend	match	london	wednesday
paul	class	teacher	february

Can you write these sentences without any mistakes? (Don't forget punctuation ! ? . and capital letters when needed)

my friend matthew and i went to see a football match

shall we go to the cinema on saturday

thursday is my favourite Day

i liked the exhibition because There were Lots of interesting g things To see

i will be going with my family to italy on Tuesday

Mary and janet liked the Painting

maggie cooked a delicious meal on sun day

> A capital letter is needed for someone's name or a specific place

> When you're talking about yourself, I always has a capital letter

Adverbs again!

Adverbs can tell you how words are said.

Can you put in an adverb which tells you how the words could be spoken. The first one has been done for you:

The dog barked loudly.

Some adverbs you could use: loudly, sadly, quietly, excitedly (already in text)

I can hear a noise upstairs. Jane said ....

We will go out later Peter said ....

I don't want to go Karim said ....

What parts of speech do they help? I know! They tell you **how, when** and **where** actions take place

Here's some more:

Adverbs can tell you how and when the things are happening.

He likes to swim frequently.

He always walks to school.

I will come over tomorrow.

I will arrive early next week.

Can you point to the adverb in these sentences?

Jason likes to work hard.

I can hear the baby upstairs.

Nina swam hard to get to the boat.

She knocked earlier than I expected.

Dad came home earlier today.

Jackie always does her homework.

He was completely tired out.

The paper arrives daily.

Can you think of the right adverbs to finish these sentences?

'Come here!' the teacher said ......

'Look what I've found!' Sharon said ......

'I've found 50p!' Felix said ......

'I will help you' the lady said ......

This rain is awful' Beatrice said ......

'I don't want to go to school' Chris said ....

Commas

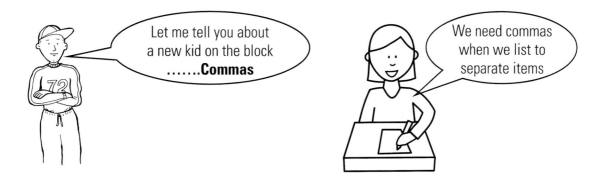

Using 'and' in a list

I need to get new socks, shoes **and** trousers. Notice the **and**

You always put **and** when it comes to the last item.

I wanted Jane, Rebecca **and** Claire to come to my party.

I am going to the shop to buy milk, butter, eggs, cereal **and** biscuits.

My favourite meal is egg, chips **and** baked beans.

I like jam, marmite, peanut butter **and** chocolate spread on my toast.

Where should the commas go?

Keira was excited going to the zoo. She wanted to see elephants monkeys giraffes and wolves.

Joshua is going on holiday. Among the clothes he needs to pack are sunglasses swimming costume T-shirts shorts and sandals.

I need to go to the supermarket to get butter cheese bread and milk.

Some of the things I must remember for school are pencils notebooks rubber and ruler.

*More commas to try don't forget the **and** this time*

I am going to make a cake I need eggs butter flour milk.

My favourite meal is egg chips baked beans ketchup.

My favourite drinks are chocolate milk shake orange lemonade tea.

My favourite TV shows are East Enders Neighbours.

Strictly Come Dancing.

> Commas are used for lists and there is always **and** before the last thing on the list.

Plurals

The easy way to show there is more than one is to **add an 's' at the end of the word**.

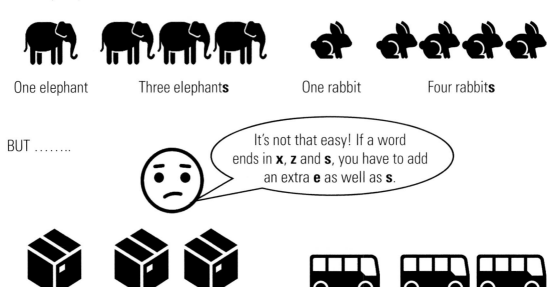

One elephant   Three elephant**s**   One rabbit   Four rabbit**s**

BUT ……..

It's not that easy! If a word ends in **x**, **z** and **s**, you have to add an extra **e** as well as **s**.

One box   Two box**es**   One bus   Two bus**es**

One kiss   Many kiss**es**   One buzz   Several buzz**es**

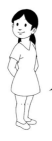

They are not the only words you need to add an **e** to the **s** to make plurals.

Words ending in **ch** and **sh** need an **e** as well as **s**.

     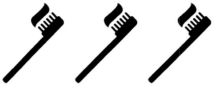

One brush   Three brush**es**

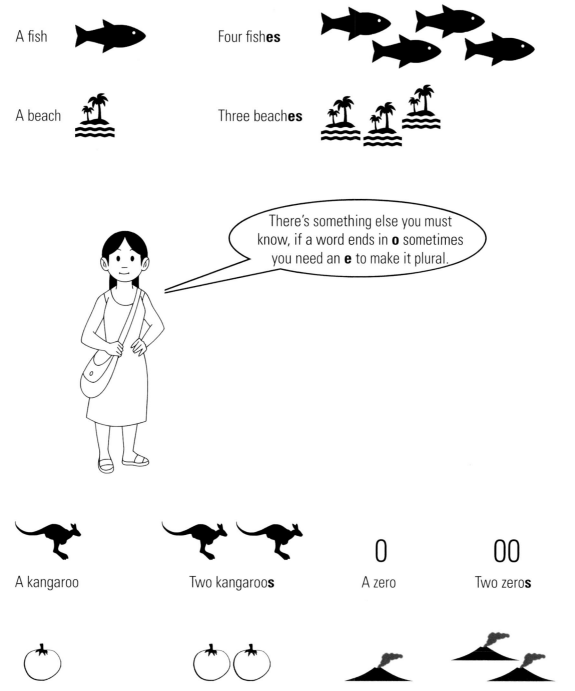

Can you make these words plural?

Singular	Plural		Singular	Plural		Singular	Plural
Cake			Church	_____		Kiss	_____
Tree			Branch	_____		Dish	_____
Frog			Glass	_____		Banana	_____
Bus			Studio	_____		Bush	_____

Commas, again!

They move upwards and become an apostrophe **' an apostrophe**

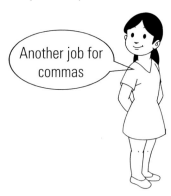

Another job for commas

Apostrophes show that something belongs to someone.

Peter's blue jacket		Jane's cat		Joanna's new car

The blue jacket belongs to Peter   This is Jane's cat   The new car belongs to Joanna

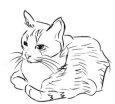

> Adding an **'s** to the end of the owner's name means it belongs to them.

The apostrophes have been left out, can you put them in?

I borrowed my sisters dress and shoes for Pamelas birthday party.

Her mothers cake looks delicious.

I used my friends laptop yesterday.

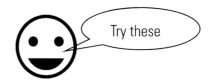

Tip: There are three of them

Here's an example:

The coat which belongs to mother is hanging in the hall

Mother**'s** coat is hanging in the hall

Try these

Can you put an apostrophe in these sentences to make them shorter?

The dog which belongs to Lita is over there.

The pie that mother baked looks wonderful.

These are the sisters called Jessica and Rita which belong to Jane.

The shoes that belong to Jessica got very wet.

Tariq has a new car which is blue.

My friend has a cat his name is Basil.

The ice cream Silda has looks delicious.

The dress Tania has is pretty.

Pesky punctuation ! ? '

 Let's look again... Revision time

How many mistakes can you find in my punctuation?

Jason loved the Seaside, He ran towards the sea with his Bucket! He collected six shells six round pebbles two pieces of seaweed?

He was cross that he had not brought his Spade with him? He would have Loved to have made a sandcastle? Suddenly he saw keith from school and borrowed keiths spade. They had a wonderful Time playing Together,

---

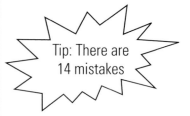

Tip: There are 14 mistakes

A reminder about plurals

One pen   Three ......

One duck   Three ....

One brush   Two ......

The fox is in the garden.   Two .... are in the garden

Can you change the words underlined into plurals and write them in the sentences?

I don't like the <u>quiz</u>.

The <u>beach</u> is quiet in the winter.

My grandma has a lovely <u>broach</u>.

My jumper is ruined after one <u>wash</u>.

I didn't like that quiz at school.
I like watching lots of ...... on television.

The ...... are quiet in the winter.

My grandma has many lovely ......

My jumpers are ruined after two ......

Still more to learn about plurals:

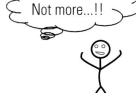
Not more...!!

For words ending in a consonant such as lady, baby, etc. get rid of the **'y'** and add **'ies'**

One lady   Three lad**ies**   A city   Three cit**ies**

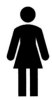 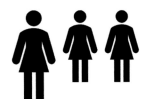

Can you choose the right spelling? Remember the rules:

We went to some good partys/parties on holiday.

There are lots of beautiful churches/churchs in the city.

We are waiting for supplys/supplies.

The flies/flys are on the wall.

I will buy lots of dresses/dresss in the sales.

The baby/babies cried loudly.

Our allotment has lots of tomatoes/tomatos.

We must pack the boxes/boxs tonight.

I'm ok with adding an **s** but I must remember it's **es** when a word ends in **ss zz o x**!

When a word ends with **y** it's **ies**.

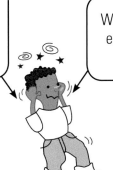

For making more than one – plurals – which words do you:

1. Just add an **s**

2. Add an **es**

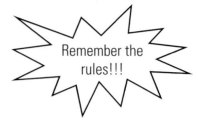

Remember the rules!!!

3. Add **ies**

Tomato ....   Daddy ....   Baby ....   Fly ....   Party ....

Box ....   Fox ....   Poppy.........   Cat ....   Kiss ....

Chose three of the plurals and write a sentence.

Opposites

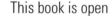

An elephant is big, a mouse is small.

Fire is hot   Ice is cold   This book is open   This book is closed

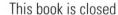

You can also make an opposite word by adding **'un'** to words.

This face is happy   This face is **un**happy

These people are being kind   These people are being **un**kind

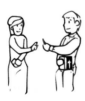
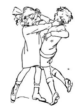

Compound words

Two words put together.

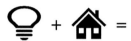
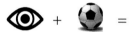

Here are some more compound words:

arm + chair = armchair   butter + fly = butterfly   rain + bow = rainbow

Can you match the right compound word to the pictures?

snowman	sunflower	ladybird
fingernail	lighthouse	eyeball

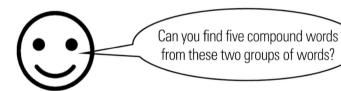

❄ + 🧍 =   ✍ + 🔩 =   💡 + 🏠 =

☀ + ✿ =   🧍 + 🐦 =   👁 + ⚽ =

Can you find five compound words from these two groups of words?

(tap) (play) (time)   (shop) (ear) (ring)

(ground) (room) (door)   (drum) (glass) (plug)

Prefix

Un added at the beginning of a word is called a **PREFIX**.

Add **un** to any of these words so they mean the opposite.

dry   pack   shout   tidy   sure   kind   city

Un at the beginning g of a word is called a **prefix**.

Adding un to words at the beginning gives the opposite meaning

The team were..........lucky to lose the match.

He felt ....well yesterday.

Jonathan's handwriting is very ......tidy.

Can you add the prefix **un** *to these words and make a sentence for each one?*

| wrap | healthy | tidy | well |

Suffix

Er added at the end of a word is called a **SUFFIX.**

Suffixes are used to compare two things: Cold Cold**er**

Tonight is *cold,* but last night it was **colder**.

Cold is the root word **er** is added to compare it.

> **er** is used to compare one against the other. It is added to the main word (the root word).

Bill is a *small* cat, but Jake is **smaller**.

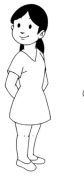 *Small* is the root word.

Chis can run *fast,* but Jake can run **faster**.

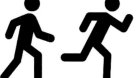 *Fast* is the root word.

Jane is *young*, but Elisabeth is **younger**.

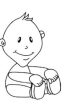

I think I am *clever*, but my sister is **cleverer**.

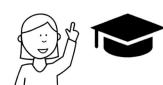

Can you finish the sentences and underline the root word (the main word)?

She comes to school late, but I am …… than she is.

My bed is soft, but Jane's is …… than mine.

Your coat is light but mine is …… than yours.

The Sun was bright yesterday but today it is ……

The water is shallow but near the rock it is ……

John is strong but Matthew is ……

It's dark in the cave, but the long tunnel is ……

Verbs and tenses

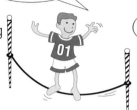

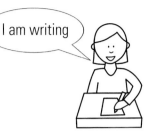

When you are talking about what is happening **now** – the simple present tense.

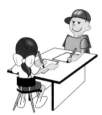

Bill and Suzanna are doing homework.

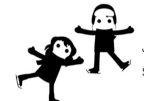

Julius and Martha are skating.

The children who are writing, doing homework, exercising, skating are all doing these things **NOW** – the present.

> You are at school now.

So when you are saying 'I am writing'
'I am exercising' you are using the present tense – called the simple present.

When it is finished, you talk in the simple past:

I was at school	I was writing	I was waiting
We were skating	We were doing homework	

Often you add **ed** at the end of a verb to move it from the present to the past.

I play tennis. I play**ed** tennis yesterday.

I talk quickly. I talk**ed** quickly.

I work at the office. I work**ed** at the office.

*Can you add **ed** to the verbs to put them in the simple past and match the picture to the verb?*

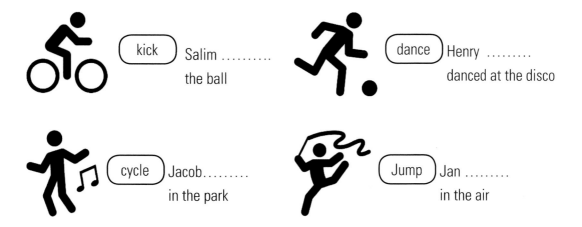

(kick) Salim .... the ball	(dance) Henry .... danced at the disco
(cycle) Jacob......... in the park	(Jump) Jan .... in the air

Can you put these verbs into the correct shape?
There are two which are a little different so be careful!

Yell	Walk**ed**	Yell**ed**
Grab	Pull**ed**	Go
Went	Eat	Hug
Ate	Growl**ed**	Kiss
Pull	Kiss**ed**	Walk
Hugged	Went	
Growl	Walk**ed**	

Simple Present

Simple Past

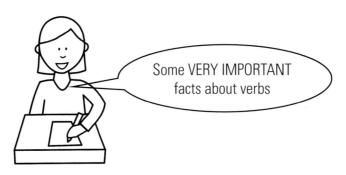

Some VERY IMPORTANT facts about verbs

When you write a sentence, you **must** choose a tense and stay with it!

You can't mix up the tenses, like these:

I listen to my tapes and I watched television, this is wrong.

It should be – I listened to my tapes and watched television

I watered the garden and drink my tea, this is wrong.

It should be – I watered my garden and drank my tea

Can you make sure these sentences have kept the same tense?

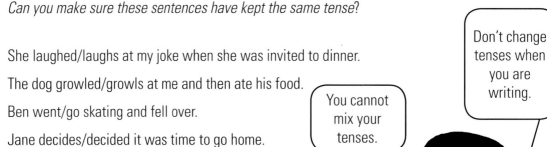

She laughed/laughs at my joke when she was invited to dinner.

The dog growled/growls at me and then ate his food.

Ben went/go skating and fell over.

Jane decides/decided it was time to go home.

The boys stay/stayed at home and watch/watched a film.

You cannot mix your tenses.

Don't change tenses when you are writing.

Can you write these sentences with the right tenses?

My cat likes to go outside hunted for mice.

Ben went swimming and dives into the deep end.

Jack plays football and scored five goals.

The dog chased the cat and it runs up the tree.

Mike enjoyed the film he laughs all the time.

BUT   There is always something which goes against the rules….

Not all present tense verbs are easy to put into the past tense by adding on **ed**.!!

Here are some of the exceptions:

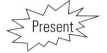

Present

Past

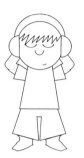

Present	Past
The bird flies	The bird flew (We don't say the bird flied)
I drink milk every day	I drank milk every day (not I drinked)
Jack runs every day	Jack ran every day (not Jack runed)
My dad drives me to school	My dad drove me to school (not dad drived)
We can hide from you	We hid from you (not we hided)
We can begin our work now	We began our work yesterday (not can begined)

Joining sentences together – another way

We have learnt about commas being used to make a list and put words together. Now we are learning how to put sentences together to make them more interesting.

Joining together with **'and'**.

Thomas likes sausages. Thomas likes chips. Joining them together

> Thomas likes sausages and chips

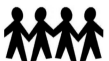

Jane is going on holiday. She is taking her swimming costume. Joining them together.

> Jane is going on holiday and she is taking her swimming costume

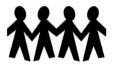

Can you join these two sentences?

I want to go to France. I want to go to Italy.

I don't like carrots. I don't like cabbage.

I watch Transformers.

I watch Star Wars.

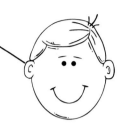

You use '**and**' to join sentences together when both ideas are as important.

Another way of joining sentences is using  **but**

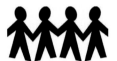

I would like to go to Germany. I do not want to go to France.

I would like to go to Germany, but I don't want to go to France.

You use '**but**' when there is an excuse or when you want to bring in another idea.

I had my homework ready. I forgot to put it in my bag.

I had my homework ready, but I forgot to put it in my bag.

Can you join these sentences together?

I wanted to take my dog for a walk. I was too tired.

Jan wants to go out. She feels ill.

I can't meet you by the park. I can meet you at the station.

Patrik had to do his homework. He wanted to play on the X box.

Another way of joining

You use **or** when it means making a choice

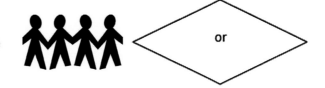

You can have milk. You can have coffee.

You can have milk **or** you can have coffee.

You can go to the cinema. You can watch television.

You can go to the cinema **or** you can watch television.

*Can you join these sentences together using **or?***

You can have chocolate.	You can have fruit.
You can go swimming.	You can play on the X box.
You can go fishing.	You can play golf.
You can go to the beach.	You can play tennis.

| Can you join these sentences using either **and, or, but**? |

I don't like sport . . . . my brother loves it.

My sister wants a puppy . . . . . . I want a cat.

We can go for a walk . . . . it's raining.

Shall we bring biscuits for Tom . . . . some cake for Beth?

I haven't decided if I want my dinner early . . . . I might prefer it later.

'You had better go inside . . . . you will catch cold' mother said.

'You can take all these things inside . . . . don't forget the plates.'

We can eat at home . . . . we can go out to a restaurant.

Remember we used the suffix **er** when comparing one against the other: My friend is tall**er** than I am

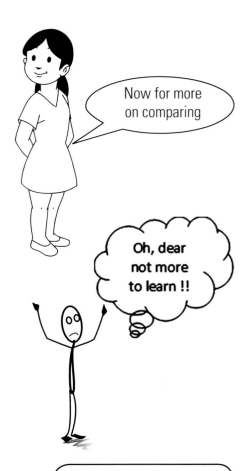

Now for more on comparing

Oh, dear not more to learn !!

This cat is small.   This rabbit is smaller.

| Comparing one against the other we use the suffix **er**. | **BUT** | When comparing more than two people or things you use **est** at the end of the word. |

Geoff is strong**er** than his friend Mark.   Mark can shout loud**er** than Matthew.

My friend is the tall**es**t in the class. (my friend is being compared to everyone in the class)

Mark can run the fast**est** in the team. (Mark can run faster than anybody in the team)
These are adjectives and are called

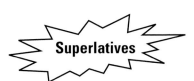

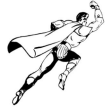

Can you put the correct comparative adjective in these sentences?
(In other words, choose either **er** or **est**)

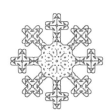 January is the …. month.   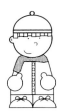 I am warm ……….. than you!

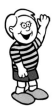 Jon is the …. boy in the class.   Jack feels …. than Frederick.

 Jonathan is the ……………. boy in the school.

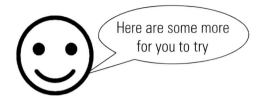

Here are some more for you to try

| thinner/thinnest happier/happiest |
| warmer/warmest   colder/coldest |
| faster/fastest sadder/saddest |

Blackberries are .... than lemons.   sweeter/sweetest

Lemons are the .... fruit.   sourer/sourest

Jake is .... than Peter.   taller/tallest

It is .... today.   colder/coldest

This pencil is the .... in the class.   newer/newest

Jane is the .... in the school.   nicer/nicest

Can you write four sentences of your own using superlatives?

Another job for the apostrophe!

Apostrophes can join two words together by replacing the missing letter or letters. It pushes them together.

You are You're ⇨ ⇦ You are

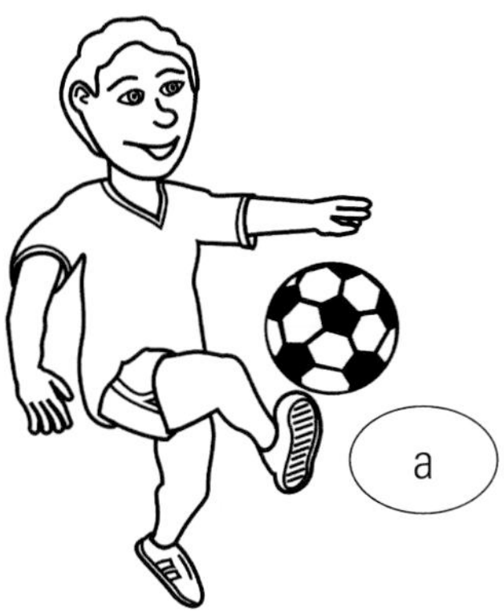
a

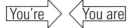

The '**a**' is kicked away!

Getting rid of the '**a**' is a more realistic way of showing when people are talking.

Look at the way these two are talking ....

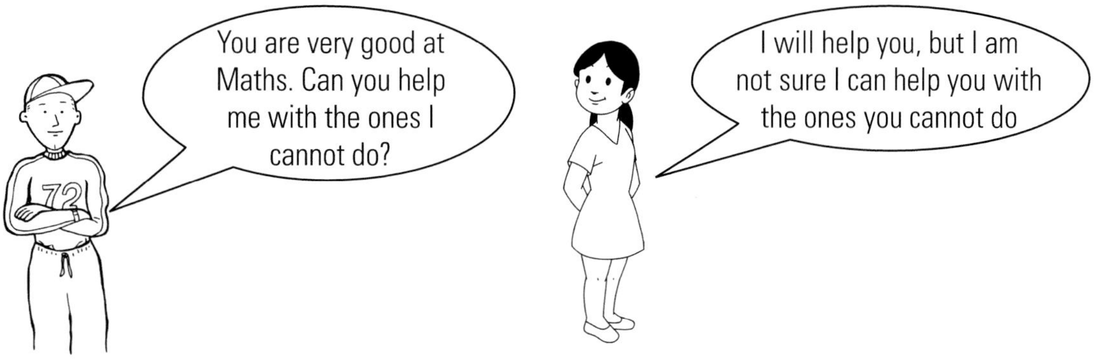
You are very good at Maths. Can you help me with the ones I cannot do?
I will help you, but I am not sure I can help you with the ones you cannot do

The talking is not very true to life. In real life they would say:

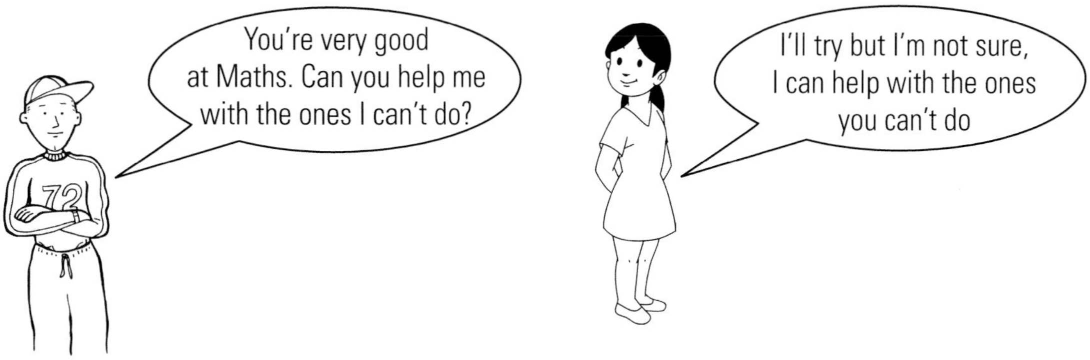
You're very good at Maths. Can you help me with the ones I can't do?
I'll try but I'm not sure, I can help with the ones you can't do

This time two letters are kicked out

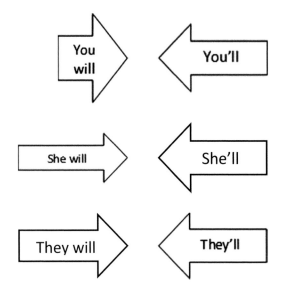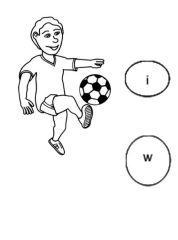

The letter '**o**' has been kicked out

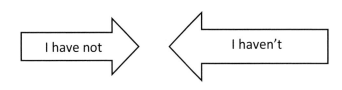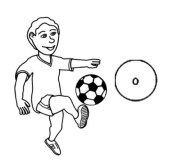

Which is the correct one?

I havent/have'nt/haven't seen the new film.

She is very late, and I can't/cant/cant' wait.

The oil is hot dont/don't/do'nt/ touch it.

I can't find my wallet it isnt'/isn't/isnt' where I left it.

Join these words together using an apostrophe

She is not ....   She is ....

Do not ....   Is not ....

Where is the phone? ....

Choose the correct one from these pairs and put them in a sentence

Couldn't	Could'nt	Wheres'	Where's
Wouldn't	Wouldnt'	Hadn't	Hadnt'

Another way of joining sentences!

We can also join sentences with

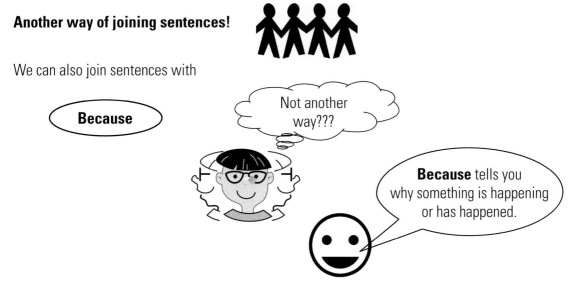

Because

Not another way???

Because tells you why something is happening or has happened.

Elena ran to school. Elena was late for school.

Elena ran to school **because** she was late – tells you **why** she ran to school.

Jason was in trouble at school. He left his homework at home. Jason was in trouble at school **because** he left his homework at home – tells you **why** he was in trouble at school.

I like football. Football is fun.

I like football **because** it's fun.

The three bears were angry. Goldilocks had eaten their porridge.

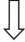

The three bears were hungry **because** Goldilocks had eaten their porridge.

I had some water. I was thirsty.

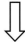

I had some water **because** I was thirsty.

Patrick ran out of the classroom. He didn't want to be late for games.

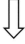

Patrick ran out of the classroom **because** he didn't want to be late for games.

Can you join these sentences with because?

I like to go to the cinema. I like to watch cartoons.

Why must I take an umbrella? It's raining now.

Why is the Sun so low in the sky? It's wintertime.

Finn must not eat too many sweets. It's not good for his teeth.

 Revision again

> You use **because** to answer the question why?

Remember joining words

> **and or because but**

Can you put in the correct one to join the sentences together?

I like John .... he doesn't like me.

I want to go to see my friend .... we have fun together.

I want to go out .... I haven't finished my homework.

My father is a doctor .... my mother is a teacher.

I like Saturdays .... I can play football.

I like to eat fish .... chips.

Jason washed the car .... it was dirty.

Jack ate all the chocolate biscuits ...... they are his favourite.

You can have ice cream .... fudge cake.

I lost your ball .... I kicked it over the fence.

I went to Spain .... France for my holidays.

You can play crazy golf .... go on the swings.

> What a lot to remember! I must keep practising ....

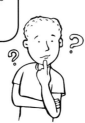

> This will remind you of what to do.

Useful words

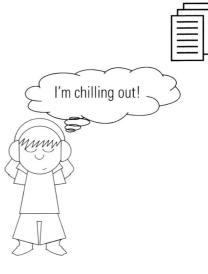

I'm chilling out!

Nouns: These are naming words. For example: table, chair, footballer.

Adjectives: They tell you more about the noun. For example: **pretty** dress, **blue** ball.

Verbs: They tell you what a person is doing. For example: John is **running** Clare is l**aughing.**

Adverb: It tells you more about the verb. For example: John ran **quickly** – how the person is running. Clare laughed **loudly** – how the person is laughing.

Capital letter: A capital letter must be at the beginning of a sentence.

You also use capital letters when you're talking about yourself. John went to the park but **I** went swimming.

You also use it when you are talking about people, days of the week, places such as London, Wednesday.

Full stop: Always have a full stop at the end of a sentence.

Commas: These needed when you have a list, apples, pears, potatoes and chocolate, BUT the last item always has *and* not a comma.

Noun phrase: These are a group of words with a noun and perhaps an adjective which tells you more about the noun. For example: A huge box.

Exclamation: A mark used when you feel strongly about something. For example: **Come here!**

Question mark: It is used at the end of questions. For example: What do you want to do**?**

Simple past tense: It tells about something that has happened in the past. For example: Jane **worked** hard.

Simple present tense: It tells about something that is happening now. For example: Jane **works** hard.

Key Stage 2 - English

Nouns

In Key Stage 1, we learnt about nouns, naming words – those that had to have a capital letter as in someone's name or a place and those that only needed them at the beginning of a sentence.

I think Mark and Paul will come with us to Scotland.

The beach was beautiful.

Nouns without a capital letter are called

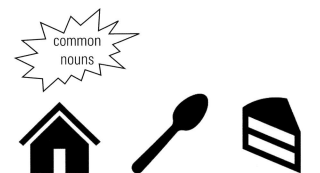

Common nouns are words you come across every day like house, spoon, cake.

Can you think of at least ten common nouns?

Remember proper nouns?

They are the names of places, people and things and they ALWAYS need a CAPITAL LETTER.

April	Brighton Beach	Thursday
Stacey	Queen Mary	Germany

So far I know about common and proper nouns but there are more . . .

Collective nouns

These are for groups of things; collective nouns are used when there are many people or things.

It sounds better than repeating 'lots of......'

A flock of sheep   A team of cyclists

A class of children   A group of dancers

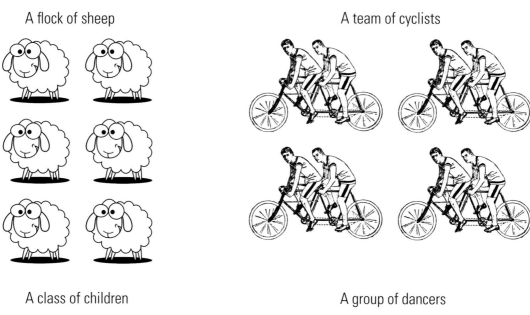

There are many more collective nouns, here are some examples:

A crowd of people   A gaggle of geese   A swarm of bees

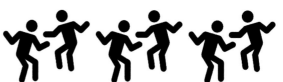

Can you think of some more?

Write out the nouns from these sentences and say if they are common, proper or collective.

In April, the beautiful flowers come out and we can hear the birds sing.

The class were very noisy during wet play on Wednesday.

We were frightened when the swarm of bees came near us.

I like to go to Hyde Park on a weekday.

There was a crowd of people by Victoria Station.

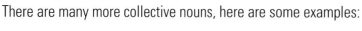

Apostrophes

Remember them?   We use apostrophes to put two words together.

We kick out the letter or letters we didn't need and put in ' instead.

I do not know where we are going.

I don't know where we're going.

Some more:

| I have | I've | I will | I'll | We are | We're | Let us | Let's |

The posh word for kicking out letters we don't need is **Contraction**.

Don't ever use an apostrophe when you are talking about more than one of anything.

You never say - I have two cats'

It should be - I have two cats

You do **not** say

Four shops'	**but**	Four shops
Five balloons'		Five balloons
Seven dogs'		Seven dogs

Never use an apostrophe when writing about more than one thing

Can you write out sentences with the right apostrophes?

Ive' gone down downstairs to look after my three cats'. I know theyre' hungry so I decided to get ten tins' of special cat food. The cats' love it!

Today Mikes' dad is taking him to see Spurs'. Hes so excited its' his first time and hes' sure th'eyll win.

Another reminder about what we've learned about the apostrophe…

We use it to show possession – in other words stuff or people they call their own.

John's dad   Peter's bike   Mum's car   My bike's saddle   The cat's basket

So far, I know apostrophes show that things or people belong to.

You also use an apostrophe to show the missing letter/letters when we join two words together.

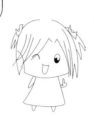

Prefixes

When we put this in front of a word it changes the meaning (**un** means not)

Remember the **prefix** **un** ?

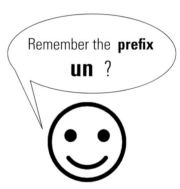

Devi was happy because his team won 6 - 0.

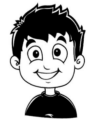

Jason was **un**happy because he lost his new Transformer model.

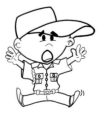

Here are more prefixes:

Re means to do something again so **re**apply means to apply again.

Mr Jones had to **re**apply the paint because it was too thin.

The house fell down and needed to be **re**built.

Pre means you've done something before.

I **pre**paid the bill   (I've paid the bill already).

You go to **pre**school before going to 'big' school.

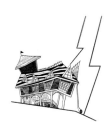

Which is the right prefix?

….heat the house please I'm still cold.

Please make sure you ….pay the hotel costs, I won't have any money.

I feel so ….happy I lost the match.

We were lucky to be able to …view the film.

This story is so ….believable.

Can you …. book the meeting I'm busy on Monday.

Mis means wrong

John **mi**sspelt many of the words.

Peter **mi**sbehaved in class and was in trouble.

Tabul X
Boook X
Pensil X

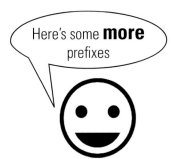
Here's some **more** prefixes

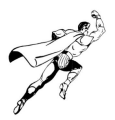

Dis means not/no

Martin and Jane **dis**agreed and started to fight.

Jake **dis**appeared before mum found about the television, he'd broken.

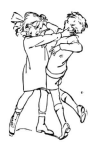

Super means greater

We love watching **super**heroes on TV.

Mum and I like shopping in our **super**market.

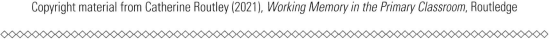

Which is the right prefix?

John......obeyed his mum so he was sent to bed.

I think Stormzy is a ....star.

'Stop......behaving' Mrs. James told Simon.

The museum has the bones of many ......historic animals.

More of those commas!

Remember we have learnt to use commas in a list, here's a reminder:

Mum went to the supermarket to get eggs, butter, chips, pizza and ketchup.

But we also use commas to show when someone is speaking. We call them speech marks and they go around the words when someone starts to speak, which is known as direct speech.

Nick said, "Cats are my favourite pets."

> Always use a capital letter when someone starts to speak.
>
> Speech always begins and ends with a punctuation mark and speech marks.

There are **3** new things to remember:

1. Speech marks when someone starts and finishes talking.

2. Use a capital letter at the beginning of the words.

3. Remember punctuation at the end – could be a . **? !**

(capital letter)   (punctuation)

"Come over here!" shouted the teacher.

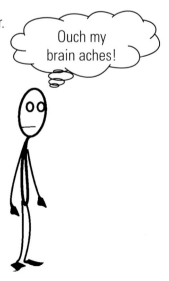

Ouch my brain aches!

Speech marks

Can you write out these sentences with the correct punctuation?

be quiet all of you yelled the policeman

will you do as you are told mum asked

You also need a **comma** before **speech** starts:

Jason said, "I would like a choc ice"

Jasmine asked, "Can I go to play now?"

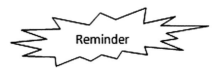

Reminder

Can you write these sentences out with capital letters and full stops?

my dog is called buster

tomorrow is my mother's birthday and

we will be going out for a super meal in london

you can get a flight from paris to london in one hour

Can you match each sentence to the correct punctuation mark?

You look fantastic	.
I can help you now	!
Where shall we go on Monday	.
I think we can see him on Sunday	!
He looks dreadful	?

Can you put some more punctuation in these sentences? Don't forget speech marks!

The chef said I am going to make a wonderful delicious casserole

Justin shouted out take care its dangerous over there

Jocelyn asked which train do I catch to go to liverpool

Compound words

They are two words joined together.

It's just a posh name for two words joined together to make a new word.

arm   +   chair

 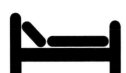   =   armchair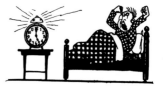

bed   +   room   =   bedroom

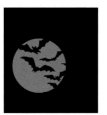

moon + light = moonlight

Some more compound words:

Hand + writing = Handwriting

Milk + shake = Milkshake

Cup + cake = Cupcake

Fire + man = Fireman

Farm + yard = Farmyard

Dish + washer = Dishwasher

Super + man = Superman

Can you make five compound words from each list:

paint	pot	rain	store
note	drop	gold	bow
snow	flake	book	cream
rain	brush	ice	fish
flower	book	star	bow

Adjectives

Adjectives make nouns more interesting – they describe the noun

The <u>hot</u> sun shone down on us   I love <u>spicy</u> food   My cat is <u>furry</u>

You can have more than one adjective to tell you about a noun. If you have more, it makes your sentence more interesting as it tells you other details about the person or thing. You can make a little list and use a comma like you did for the shopping.

The brave, strong soldier   The beautiful, furry kitten   A cold, dark night

Circle the adjectives in the below given sentences

The dark, winding path led to the old house.

Martin saw the miserable, crumbling hut deep in the creepy, dark wood.

The old, battered door was open and banged against the rotten frame.

The boys didn't know what to do. They were cold, frightened children.

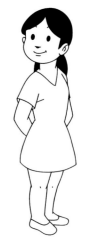

I can easily spot an adjective, it's always before the noun

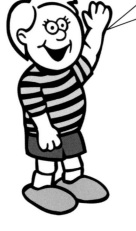

No, that's not always so! They can come after the noun

	Noun	Adjective	Adjective

The knight's armour was heavy and uncomfortable

Joan's coat was warm and colourful.   Peter's dog was fierce and ugly.

Can you put your own adjectives in these sentences?

The .... snow covered the .... valley and the .... children made their way along the........ path.

Jennifer wanted to go to the .... swimming pool and packed her ......, ... swimming costume.

The .... teacher was very cross with the ...., ... class and told them so in a .... voice.

Synonyms

That's a word which has similar, or almost
the same meaning as another. Similar sounds a little like
synonym which makes it easy to remember.

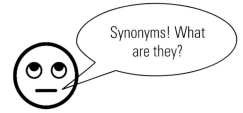

Using synonyms for everyday words makes it more interesting. Instead of using kind/said/
frightened/walk try these:

Synonyms for **kind**
gentle   thoughtful
considerate   attentive

Synonyms for **said**
added   announced
continued   observed

Synonym for **frightened**
afraid   scared   terrified   horrified

Synonyms for **walk**
wander   trudge   stroll
trek   amble

Can you write three sentences with synonyms for
1) walk   2) kind   3) said

Replace the words underlined with another one from the list below

delighted   furious   tasty   dazzling   courageous   miserable

I had a delicious sandwich for lunch yesterday.

Dad was angry when someone crashed into his car.

Jennifer was sad when the party finished.

Sita was happy to go to the cinema.

The bride looked beautiful.

The policeman was very brave when he stopped the criminal.

Pronouns

You use pronouns instead of nouns – it stops you repeating the noun and making the sentence too long and boring.

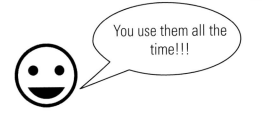

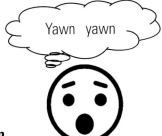

There are different types of pronouns:

Kate said **she** would bring the cakes to the party, but she forgot **them**.

      She replaces the name Kate. **Them** is a pronoun that replaces cakes.

Jack and **I** wanted to see the film, so **we** booked **it** for Monday.

      We is a pronoun replacing Jack and I. **It** is a pronoun replacing the film.
(It would be very long and boring if we said 'Jack and I wanted to see the film, so Jack and I booked the film for Monday')

Jon and Mo were told off by the teacher. **They** had to stay in playtime.

      They is instead of Jon and I.

Can you point to the pronouns in the following sentences?

You and I can see him on Friday.

He wanted to repair the car.

Let's go and see them tomorrow.

We can see her soon.

We can do this ourselves without your help.

Let's go to her house on Monday.

Can you make these sentences shorter and not so boring by using pronouns for the words underlined?

Lila and Patrick were going to see the show on Friday, Lila and Patrick wanted to see the show for ages.

Graham was tired and hungry when he got home. Graham ate a huge supper.

Peter is a clever boy. Peter enjoys school very much.

Kevin and Paul had a tennis match. Kevin and Paul were good tennis players. Kevin and Paul like to play tennis every week.

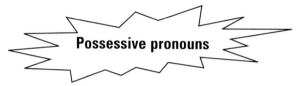

Possessive pronouns

This is just a posh name for pronouns which show who owns something like

mine   yours   ours   his/her   their

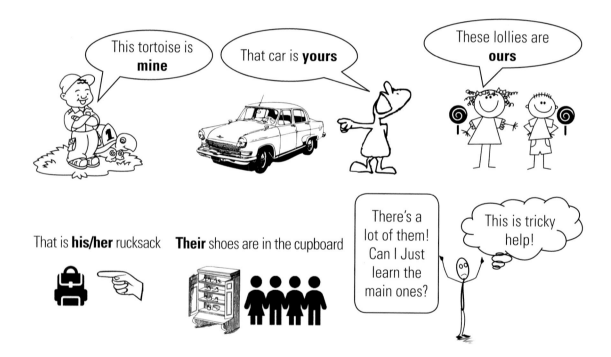

You use these pronouns if the person or thing is doing the action.

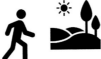

He walked to the park.

They waited for the train.

The bird was frightened, it flew away.

We use these when the action is being done to a group of people or things.

We told **them** to do the work   I'm taking **them** to the cinema   I will invite **them** to my party

The boys were hungry, so Mum gave **them** some ice creams

Can you put the right pronouns in these sentences?

George and Tim were very hot so .... both went swimming.

Petra and Liam had lost their sports gear so .... decided to search the changing rooms.

Jacob loves building things, ... favourite toy is Lego.

Susie, Alison and Nell just missed the train so .... had to wait for another hour.

'No' these places are .... said Jen 'we saved them for our friends'.

The little boy shouted. 'that is ....' as he snatched the toy car.

'Please give Jeanette .... Sindy doll back' said Mum.

Remember adverbs?

We learned that adverbs tell you more about verbs they tell you when, where and how something is done.

Here's some you recognise:

He walked quickly – quickly tells you how he walked, it is the adverb.

John climbed the ladder safely – safely tells you how John climbed.

We learned:

1. Adverbs don't have to end in **ly**.

Matthew was upstairs – upstairs tells you where Matthew was.

2. Adverbs don't have always to go after the verb, they can be before the verb.

He **silently** crept up the stairs

One thing we haven't learned is that

Perhaps, I will see the show

Usually, I see him on a Monday

Afterwards, we can have a meal

Can you put in an adverb for these sentences?

I was so pleased Jennifer came over .... to see us.

.... he ran up the stairs.

He crept .... up the stairs.

He can't hear you he is .... in his bedroom.

Go away! The lady shouted ....

The man shouted .... at the waiter.

The fox .... followed the hen.

The giant .... burst into the room.

> Oh, dear I must think again about the job of an adverb

> Adverbs can be at the **beginning** of a sentence

| angrily | silently | noisily | yesterday |
| furiously | upstairs | cautiously | timidly |

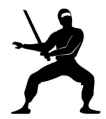

Determiners – articles

Nothing to be scared about! they are articles like **a**, **an**, **the**.

Depending on which article you use it can change the idea of the sentence

If you say

'I saw **a** witch'

It could be any witch I saw

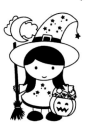

but

'I saw **the** witch'

It was a specific (special) witch

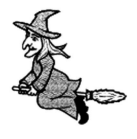

It's important that you must know:

We say and write ....

an idea   an elephant   an apple

But ...

a table   a pencil   a shop

But guess what?   ..... it's not that simple

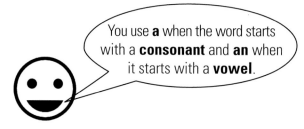

REMEMBER when to use **a** and when to use **an**

You use **a** when the word starts with a **consonant** and **an** when it starts with a **vowel**.

Some words start with a vowel but sound like they should start with consonants.

a university   a uniform   a ukulele   a unicorn

They sound as if they really start with a **y** which is a consonant, so they use 'a'

a history lesson   **a** happy person

What do you do with words starting with **h**?

If you don't actually say the **h** as in an heir to the throne, you use 'an'

an honourable man

If you *say* the **h** as in happy, history then you use **a**

Can you match a or an to these words?

......unicorn   ......alligator   ......table   ......grape

......hour   ......universe   ......ship   ......honour

......uncle   ......hotel   ......pencil   ......lesson

Verbs

So far, we have learnt about present simple and past simple. To show a verb is in the past, we add **ed**.

Present   Past

talk   talk**ed**   but surprise, surprise ......not all verbs follow that rule!!

show   show**ed**

Here are some that don't

Present	see	eat	take	think	have	do	come	speak
Past	saw	ate	took	thought	had	did	came	spoke

Write out the sentences that are in the past tense

Jennifer thought she would go to the park.

Jack jumps extremely high.

He drank lots of milk.

Pauline eats a lot of food.

Patrick danced all night.

He spoke to the teacher.

I think she is horrible.

He came to the pool on Tuesday.

He laughed out loud.

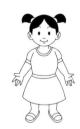

You can put **will** in front of the verb, and it puts it in the future.

If you are going to do something later, you use the **future** tense

I **will** read the book tomorrow.

I **will** cook a super meal on Friday.

I **will** swim tomorrow.

When something is going on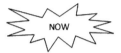

you use part of the verb (I am, you are etc) and an ing verb.

We **are going** to the cinema

We **are running** for the bus

We **are playing** football

And if it's

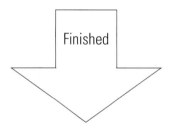

Finished

Then you use the past tense of the 'to be' verb

I was, you were, they were.

We were going home.

You were tired yesterday.

If something is going to happen, you put will in front of the verb

You use are and ing to show something is happening now

Were/was is used to show the action is finished

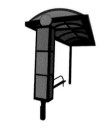

I am waiting at the bus stop.

I was waiting at the bus stop but got fed up.

Tomorrow I will be waiting at the bus stop.

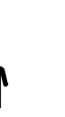

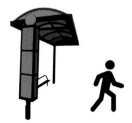

Can you make up three sentences using the verbs?

shout   follow   jump   laugh   eat

showing the action taking place in   the present   the past   the future

Those adverbs again!

A different job for the adverb – they can also describe adjectives as well as verbs!

She is **quite** pretty.

That dog is **extremely** big.

John is **very** thin.

The food is **so** delicious.

The show was **really** awesome.

They modify the adjective – they tell you more about it

Adverbs are very busy!

If an adverb tells you more about the adjective, it always comes first.

The cat's bowl is quite big.

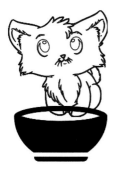

The cat's bowl is extremely big.

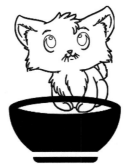

There are other adverbs that can tell you more about other adverbs......

The teacher shouted <u>really loudly</u>.   Laura waited <u>perfectly quietly</u>

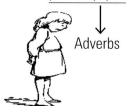

This time they tell you more about the adverb.

These words; friendly, lovely can trick you! These words
may end in **ly** but they are NOT adverbs.

The girl had a lovely dress, tells you about the dress.

The boy had a friendly smile, describes the boy's smile.

Don't think **ly** is
always an
adverb!

The lady swam daily, this is an adverb that tells you when the lady swam.

The daily newspaper is here, tells you about the newspaper.

Can you tell whether the word underlined is being used as an adverb or adjective?

He trod <u>softly</u> down the stairs   I like <u>fast</u> cars   He's a <u>hard</u> man

The teacher looked <u>angrily</u> at the child   The sweets are <u>free</u>   The man arrived <u>late</u>

The book is <u>upstairs</u> on the shelf   You need to drive <u>slowly</u>   Joe punched <u>hard</u>

Plurals again

We already know something about plurals   you add an **s**:

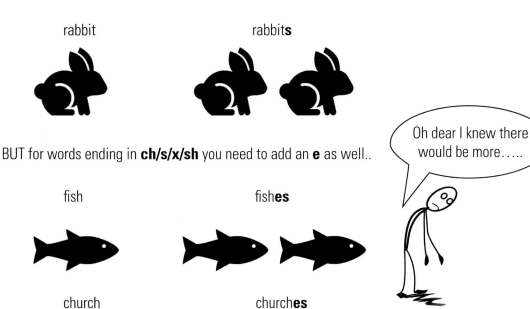

rabbit   rabbit**s**

BUT for words ending in **ch/s/x/sh** you need to add an **e** as well..

Oh dear I knew there would be more…..

fish   fish**es**

church   church**es**

Words ending in **o** have an **s** or **es** added.

tomato   tomato**es**

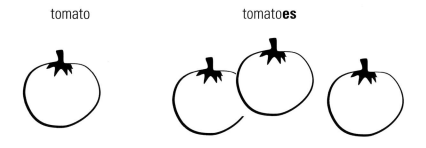

Sometimes (not always) for words ending in **y** you need to add **ies**.

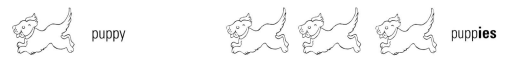

puppy   puppp**ies**

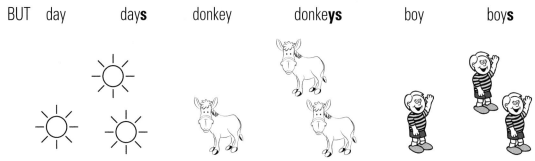

BUT   day   day**s**   donkey   donke**ys**   boy   boy**s**

Another rule:

When a word ends in **f** or **fe** you have to replace these letters with **ves** to make it plural

shelf   shel**ves**   wife   wi**ves**   knife   kni**ves**   calf   cal**ves**   leaf   lea**ves**

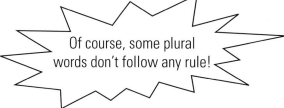

Of course, some plural words don't follow any rule!

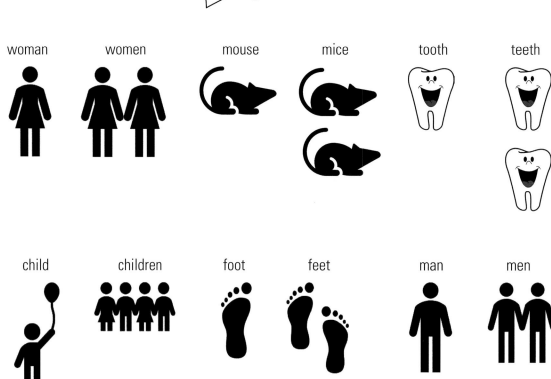

woman   women   mouse   mice   tooth   teeth

child   children   foot   feet   man   men

Back to the apostrophe

Remember, to show something belongs to someone you use an apostrophe.

The dog's ball   The rabbit's carrot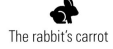

Even if a word ends in an **s** you do the same…

St Thomas's hospital is in London   Lucas's car is very smart   Marcus's house is in Bath

If something belongs to a group of people or things and ends in **s** just add the apostrophe.

Here is the dogs' food (for more than one dog)

Here is the dog's food (for one dog)

If it doesn't end in an **s** like men, women, put the apostrophe as you would a single word.

The children's toys are everywhere   The women's clothes are on the first floor

Where does the apostrophe go in the sentences below?

The puppies beds are in the kitchen.

The mans hat was under the chair.

The chefs hats are white.

My glasses case is missing.

The schools building is an old one.

The babies cries are heard all over the street.

The sheep field has a long way away.

The wolves leader was killed.

Just a reminder about the exclamation mark!

You use it when

You want to be bossy	**Come here at once!**
When someone is shouting	**Help!**
To show surprise or anger	**He's got pink hair!**

You **don't** use it at the same time as a full stop.

When it's just a statement, for example: I am going to the park today.

Write out the sentences and put in the correct exclamation marks.

She looked at Jane in amazement 'Well, you do look fantastic'

I will get the bus to town

The ghost is coming after me

Are you coming with me

I'm going to watch a boring film with my mother today

You are very stupid

I'm going to school today

Remember the pronouns?

The ones about the person or thing doing the action.

Jennifer was tired, **she** got the bus home. Matthew thought about it, **he** was going to tell the truth.

These pronouns are the ones we use when the action is being done by someone else.

They built a wonderful sandcastle. **We** will go to the beach soon.

Let's surprise **them** with a party.

Can you give **us** some idea of the time you will get here?

I told **him** the answer.

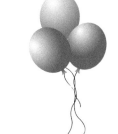

Put in the pronouns

The cake is for ......

The clock has broken we will have to throw ...... away.

The ghost chased ...... down the road.

He didn't want to tell ..... the truth.

Susanna was late ..... ran quickly to the bus stop.

Questions

We learnt about when to use question marks (?) Questions often start with a question word.

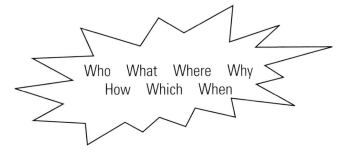

Who   What   Where   Why
How   Which   When

Who will take the dog to the park?   When can we go home?   Which one would you like?

Sometimes a statement such as: The boys want to do swimming, can be changed into a question by putting a verb at the beginning, e.g. Do the boys want to go swimming?

Statement	**Question**
We are going camping.	Are we going camping?
She is walking home	Is she walking home?
They are going out	Are they going out?
They went out	Did they go out?

Can you change these statements into a question?
(don't forget to check if the verb is in the present or past tense)

The dogs are hungry.

The cat went out.

The class was quiet.

The weather is cold today.

The boys played football.

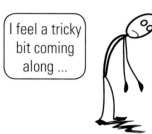

I feel a tricky bit coming along ...

Phrases and clauses

We've talked about sentences – the basic (easy) ones are made up   subject + verb + object

The <u>children</u> <u>picked</u> the <u>apples</u>.
subject   verb   object

What is a phrase?

A phrase is part of a sentence, usually without a verb, which gives you more information about the noun.

A noun = The children

The noisy children tells you more about the children

The noisy, hungry children tells you even more about the children

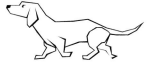

Now things are going to get slightly more difficult

The caterpillar   The slimy, tiny caterpillar   The dog   The skinny, friendly dog

Can you write noun phrases about?

A mouse   A rabbit   An ice cream

What is a clause?

A clause is a name for a part of a sentence, and it has only one verb.

I live in London   I eat chips   I like strawberries   My cat eats chicken

To make it more interesting you add a bit more with the help of a joining word – a conjunction or a pronoun.

I like strawberries because they're sweet.   I live in London which is in England.

⇩   ⇩

Conjunction   Pronoun

So, what's the difference:

A **phrase** is a part of a sentence usually without a verb which doesn't make sense on its own i.e. 'down by the stream'.

A **clause** is the part of a sentence which has a **subject** and a **verb**.

Jacob took his book.   This is a clause because it has a verb (took) and a subject (Jacob)

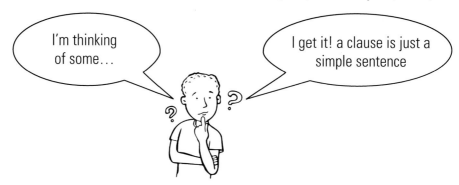

Peter likes sport, Maria hates netball   are phrases

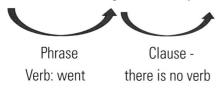

We went swimming at the local pool

Phrase
Verb: went

Clause -
there is no verb

Can you underline the phrase in these sentences? Remember: It has to have a verb

Jonathan likes to go ski boarding in the French Alps.

The meal was super especially the desert.

Jacob likes to ride his bike in the park.

The scary green monster came out of the woods.

Can you underline the clause in these sentences?

The dogs were barking in the garden.

I like to swim in the sea best.

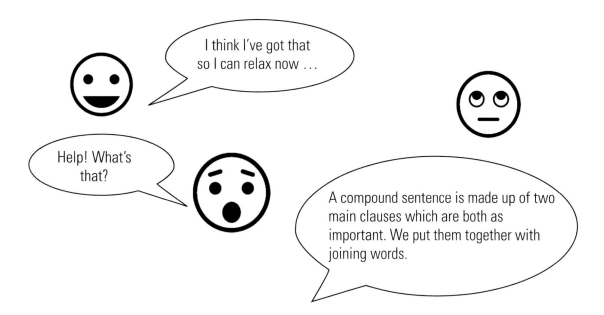

Hang on a minute, now we are going to talk about a **compound sentence**.

The family were eating their meal in the kitchen.   We enjoyed the show at the theatre.

I think I've got that so I can relax now …

Help! What's that?

A compound sentence is made up of two main clauses which are both as important. We put them together with joining words.

Joining words

We've met some of them: **and, or, but**.

These joining words make a **compound** sentence, other joining words which do the same job: **so, yet**

The dinner looked awful	**so**	I refused to eat it

main clause   connective   main clause

*Can you use these conjunctions to join these sentences together choosing from **so, yet, and, or, but**? The first one has been done for you.*

I haven't been learning for a long time, yet I can do the work.

I like coffee, ……my wife prefers tea.

I was early….we were all ready for bed after our long walk.

I have eaten three chocolate bars….I feel sick.

Would you like cake… would you …….ice cream.

John and family are very late ….they   will not be coming to dinner.

Prefixes

Remember the prefix, the bit that goes in front of a word to change the meaning.

An active cat

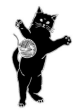

An **in**active cat

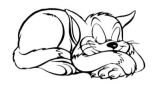

A friendly boy

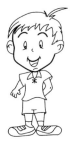

An **un**friendly boy

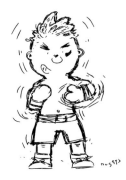

They two men agreed

The children **dis**agreed about their game

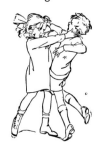

Other prefixes:

Mrs. Parker **re**planted the flowers in the garden after the rain – Mrs. Parker planted the flowers again.

He **pre**paid the bill to **pre**vent any problems means he paid the bills before.

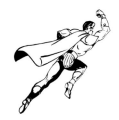

The submarine went **under** the water (it sent under the water).

Jason wants to be a **super**hero (better than your average hero).

Can you put in the correct prefix to describe?

Someone who is not friendly......... friendly.

The action the man has to do to paint the fence again   ......paint it.

Mrs. Kaur told Simon 'You are a ......star'.

The cottage fell down, so they had to... build it.

Our new teacher works so hard I would say he is ......working.

Jane is so thin she is .....weight.

I can't understand what Jason says, he talks a lot of ..... sense.

We have to ....line the heading in our books.

Homophones

These are the words that sound the same but have different meanings.

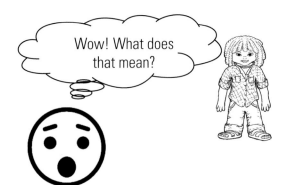

Wow! What does that mean?

Here we go.....

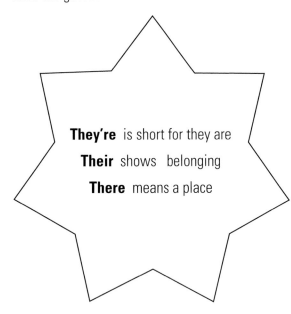

They're is short for they are

Their shows belonging

There means a place

We're	short for we are
Wear	I **wear** T shirts
Where	are my books?
	This is **where** I live
Were	We **were** going to the cinema

Match the right spelling

Can you see my purse? I left it .... | there

.... teacher is very strict

I think .... on the bridge | their

I don't like .... work

Look! it's over .... | they're

I like to .... jeans on the weekend | wear

.... is my coat? | were

This is .... I left my car

.... have I left my keys? | where

Mum and dad .... going out

.... going out now | we're

Here are some more:

brake   break   pair   pear   week   weak   great   grate   heel   heal

see   sea   knight   night   our   hour   morning   mourning   blew   blue

Can you choose the right word from the list above to finish these sentences?

The girl's dress was b.........   He felt w...... after his illness.

This is g .... house.   My h....... is sore.

The s......... is rough today.   I have a new p....... of shoes.

It's b......... time at 11 o'clock.

Suffixes

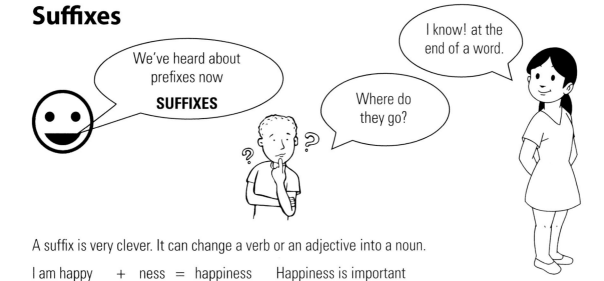

A suffix is very clever. It can change a verb or an adjective into a noun.

I am happy   + ness = happiness   Happiness is important
    adjective   noun

He needs to be punished   +   ment = punishment   He had to take his punishment
              verb   noun

Here are some more examples:

I enjoy television + ment = My <u>enjoyment</u> is watching television

Mark was sad yesterday + ness = Mark's <u>sadness</u> was most upsetting

I will teach the class tomorrow + er = The <u>teacher</u> will teach class tomorrow

Can you add the right suffix you need to make these verbs into nouns?

Tired....   Weak....   Manage....   Enjoy....   Amaze...   Retire....   Aware....

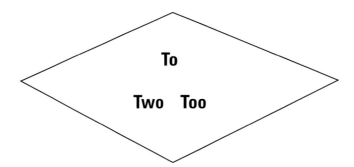

I thought we'd finished with homophones.

Some more of those words that sound the same ......   Here are some you have heard of:

To

Two   Too

To is a preposition when it comes before a noun. We are going **to** the shop. We are going to France.

It can mean going towards something or someone **to**, somewhere and it can also be part of a verb in its simplest like go **to**, walk **to**, run **to**, jump **to**.

Too can mean as well, also and too much.

Your coat is **too** big   Sita came too   We can't go out, it's **too** hot   I would like to see him **too**

Two is really easy, **it** means the number 2.   I will eat **two** hot dogs.

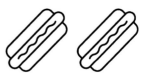

*Can you put in the right **to/two/too** in these sentences?*

His work is .... easy.

No wonder he is overweight, he eats .... much.

I don't think he wants .... come ....

I am .... busy to see you.

Can we go .... the park now?

He saw .... birds in the garden.

He ran .... the park.

Can we remember?

Which is the right pronoun to put in the sentences?

his her she him while until

Peter was listening to the radio ...... doing his homework.

Jasmin was excited ...... was going to the concert with ...... friend.

You can borrow this ...... I need it.

Matthew decided to put ...... boots on ...... waiting for ...... friend.

Philip let me use ...... car.

...... he was sleeping the dog barked loudly.

Remember synonyms and antonyms?

Synonyms

Words that mean the same or something which is very similar to another word.

Jacob's party was a wonderful surprise.

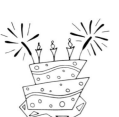

> **Synonyms** for wonderful
>
> amazing fantastic glorious tremendous
> awesome incredible

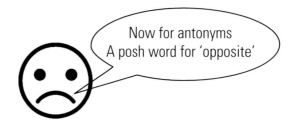

Now for antonyms
A posh word for 'opposite'

Antonyms

A word opposite in meaning to another word.

It was a dreadful day, rain all day long.   It was a **wonderful** day, sunshine all day.

Beautiful is the opposite of dreadful. In other words, it's an **antonym**.

> **Antonyms** for wonderful
> awful dreadful appalling
> horrendous nasty horrible

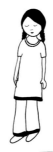

Emily felt miserable, she didn't want to go to the party.

Synonyms for miserable

mournful forlorn gloomy dejected
unhapy dejected

Antonyms for miserable

cheerful happy elated joyful
merry thrilled

The sea around the tiny island was calm.

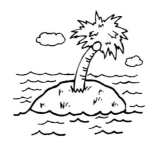

Antonyms for calm

tempestuous choppy rough stormy
turbulent

Synonyms for calm

still tranquil peaceful
serene restful

Bruno is a tiny dog but he barks loudly.

Synonyms for tiny

small little mini minute

Antonyms for tiny

huge massive colossal imposing
enormous immense

Can you put these synonyms and antonyms in the correct columns?

demanding   clear   effortless   simple   complicated   hard   exacting   unchallenging
difficult   stiff   unclear   tough   exacting   straightforward

Synonyms of easy	**Antonyms** of easy

Can you write these sentences using an antonym for the words underlined?

The Sun shone <u>brightly</u>.

Jack drove off in his <u>shinny</u> car.

The <u>skinny</u> cat walked away.

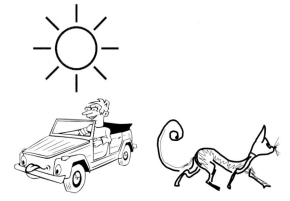

Colons

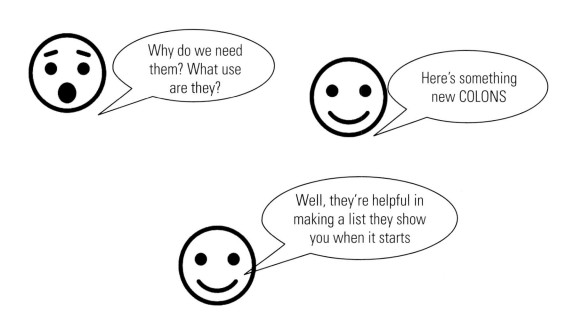

"I need lots of things for my camping trip: tent, sleeping bag, ground sheet and stove."

They are also useful when you want to go into more detail and make your sentence more interesting.

For example: I know our cat loves fighting, it has very sharp teeth.

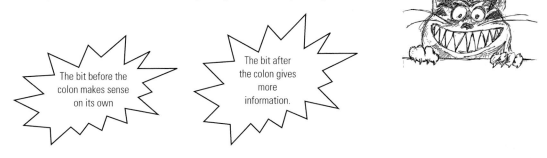

There is one country I really want to visit: Mexico (explains the main idea)

Main idea

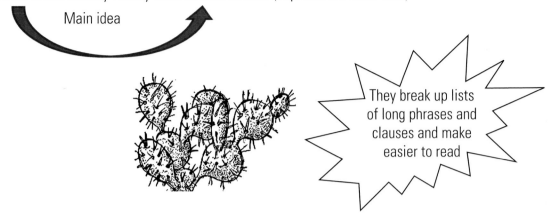

They break up lists of long phrases and clauses and make easier to read

Please copy out these sentences and add a colon in the correct place

I need these things to make a cake flour, butter and sugar.

There is just one present I would like for my birthday a pony.

Jonathan was feeling very sick he'd eaten three chocolate bars one after the other.

Seth was feeling very proud he had won the medal for the 200 metres race.

Semicolons

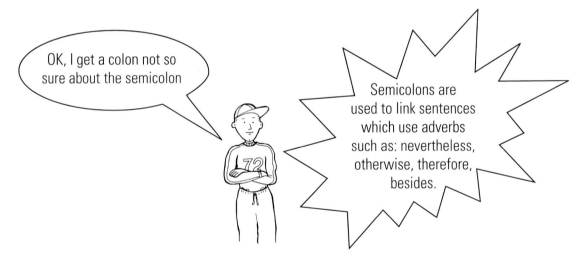

OK, I get a colon not so sure about the semicolon

Semicolons are used to link sentences which use adverbs such as: nevertheless, otherwise, therefore, besides.

Here are some examples:

When we went to Scotland, we visited lots of castles; we went to see how haggis was made; I bought some Edinburgh rock; and my sister annoyed me all the time.

I had a row with my sister; nevertheless, we still went shopping together.

They also turn two sentences into one.   BUT they must be about the same thing and have the same importance and must make sense on their own.   You could say they are *instead of a conjunction*

Here's an example:

Matthew went to the station to say goodbye to his friend *because* he wouldn't see him for ages.

Matthew went to the station to say goodbye to his friend; he wouldn't see him in ages.

Which ones do you think can be connected with a semicolon?

My mother doesn't like rice pudding......... milk doesn't agree with her.

I like Spain......... hot weather and good food.

I really wanted to go to the match......... my favourite team are playing.

My grandfather doesn't like going to bed early......... there is too much to see on television.

I want to go to the swimming pool......... our house needs painting.

My brother is going running today......... he is training for the marathon.

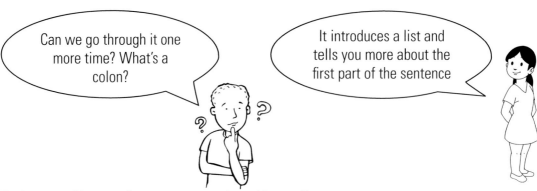

Dad was cooking our dinner: a cottage pie and broccoli.

For my salad I will need: lettuce, cucumber and tomatoes.

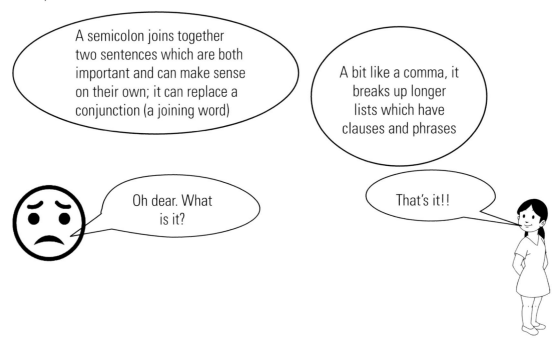

The children had a great time on the beach; they went in and out of the water; gathered pretty seashells; made sandcastles and ate lots of ice creams.

I'm not going to the Sun this year; hot Sun doesn't agree with me.

Compound sentences

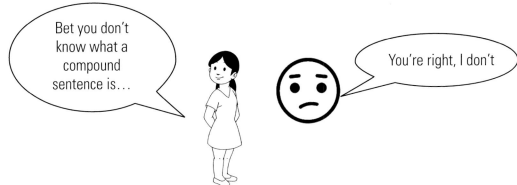

Here's some examples:

Joel collects Star Wars figures. Henry prefers dinosaur models.

Sienna wanted to go out. She was told she had to stay in.

Joel collects Star Wars figures **however** Henry prefers dinosaur models.

Sienna wanted to go out, **but** she told she had to stay in.

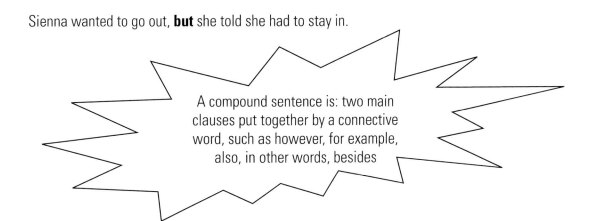

A compound sentence is: two main clauses put together by a connective word, such as however, for example, also, in other words, besides

Here are some more examples:

I watched the squirrel **until** it ran away.

He goes to lots of music festivals **although** he doesn't like music.

We went to bed **and** slept until morning.

You can watch your programme **if** you finish your homework.

He waited **until** the show finished.

Can you join these sentences choosing the best suited conjunctions from the words in the circle?

The class were playing about .... I was working hard.

She went to the film .... she had read the book.

She had hurt her ankle .... playing tennis.

Do you mind .... I sit down, I'm tired.

I can help you .... I can.

I decided to run outside .... the others were busy.

until if while
because

Useful words

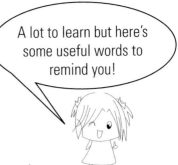

A lot to learn but here's some useful words to remind you!

Adjective: A word that describes a noun. For example:
a small cat, a hot day.

Adverb: A word that tells you more about a verb. For example:
James ran quickly; Keira walked slowly.

BUT Adverbs can also tell you more about another adjective. For example:
The cat is extremely pretty. The food was quite dreadful.

Antonym: A word which means the opposite of another. For example: The tiny dog. The huge dog.

Apostrophe: ʼ It has two jobs. 1. Shows when there are missing letter(s). For example:
Change have not into haven't, should not into shouldn't
2. Shows when something belongs to someone (it's called possession). For example: Joanne's dog, Peter's car.

Capital letters: We use them always at the beginning of a sentence and for names of people and places. For example: London, Germany, Martin, Patricia.

Clause: Part of a sentence that has groups of words that contain a subject and a verb. For example: The skinny cat ran up the tree.

Colon: : Introduces lists and joins sentences. For example: There were many exciting books in the shop: Star wars annuals, the new Harry Potter.

It can also tell you more about the first part of the sentence. For example: I have to go now: my train leaves soon.

Comma: , Has many uses: separates items in a list, joins clauses and can give extra information, separates two sentences with a conjunction. For example: Most birds have separate toes, but ducks' feet are webbed.

It can also separate parts of a sentence. Jane, hungry as she was, was too frightened to ask for food.

Conjunctions: Joins two sentences or clauses together such as and, but, so, or, however.

Compound sentence: Joins two parts of a sentence with a connective word (and, but, so but, or). For example: I like bananas and I like grapes.

Contraction: By joining two words together with an apostrophe. The word gets smaller – it gets contracted. For example: I should not becomes I shouldn't.

Determiner: A small word that goes before a noun to let you know if you talking about a special thing or in general. For example: The large cat was greedy. A large cat is greedy.

Exclamation mark: !> When someone feels strongly about something. For example: That dress is beautiful! to give an order Come here at once!

Full stop: It always goes at the end of a sentence.

Homophone: Words that sound the same but have different meanings. For example: brake and break.

Main clause: The most important bit of a sentence makes sense on its own. For example: I saw him even though it was very dark. I saw him is the main bit of the sentence (the main clause).

Phrase: A small part of a sentence which doesn't make sense on its own. For example: The small grey squirrel.

Prefix: Letters that go in front of a word to change its meaning. For example: He read the ingredients and made a delicious cake. He **mis**read the ingredients; the cake tasted dreadful.

Preposition: A word that tells you where things are. For example: above, below, in front or, behind.

Pronoun: There are two kinds of pronouns. The ones used instead of a noun. For example: I, You, he, they and the ones that show belonging you're, their, mine.

Question mark: ?> It goes at the end of a sentence. For example: Where is he?

Semicolon: Semicolons are mainly used within a sentence to separate clauses. The clauses must be related and not be joined together with a conjunction; the semicolon takes the place of the conjunction. For example: I love to sing but my brother loves to act. It could be written as I love to sing; my brother loves to act.

Suffix: Letters that can be put after a word to make a verb into a noun. For example: The work needs amending (verb). You need to make an amendment to your work (noun).

Synonym: A word with the same or close to the same meaning as another. For example: huge and enormous.

Verb: A doing word. A sentence *must* have a verb. For example: The old man sat on the seat for ages. Paul enjoyed his meal.